Wakefield Press

Seventeen Voices

Marianne Broug was a music teacher and member of the Adelaide Symphony Orchestra, whose career was interrupted by severe anxiety, panic attacks and depression. She has had a children's music book, *Flute with a Twist*, published. She is now a writer and lives in the Adelaide Hills.

Seventeen Voices

Life and wisdom from inside 'mental illness'

Marianne Broug

Wakefield Press

Wakefield Press
1 The Parade West
Kent Town
South Australia 5067
www.wakefieldpress.com.au

First published 2008

Cover designed by Liz Nicholson, designBITE
Typeset by Ryan Paine, Bovine Industries, Melbourne
Printed in Australia by Griffin Press, Adelaide

National Library of Australia
Cataloguing-in-Publication entry

Author: Broug, Marianne, 1959–   .
Title: Seventeen voices: life and wisdom from inside
                 'mental illness'/Marianne Broug.
ISBN: 978 1 86254 801 5 (pbk.).
Subjects: Mentally ill – Interviews – South Australia.
                 Mental illness – South Australia.
Dewey Number: 305.9084

Government
of South Australia

Arts SA

fox creek
wines

For the countless human beings around the world,
who day by day
endure tremendous suffering
and whose suffering is only compounded by
myths, misconceptions,
stigmas and stereotypes.

And for Frank

Contents

Acknowledgments

My deepest and most heartfelt thanks to the seventeen people who contributed to this book by giving of their time and sharing intimate aspects of their lives. My hope is that the stories of your courage, understanding and wisdom will be heard by many. Thanks also for the personal support and encouragement you have given me.

Thanks to Sharon for her steadfast encouragement and love; to Trevor Parry for his encouragement, assistance and positive outlook on the project; to Trish Parry for carrying Trevor's determination forward; to Patrick Kelly for inspiration, friendship and much-needed sanity; to Andrew Gara for his support; to Nancy Caldwell for her assistance; to Rosalie Pace for community support and assistance; to the Obsessive Compulsive Disorders Support Service Inc.; to the Panic Anxiety Disorder Association (PADA); and to the community mental health movement GROW.

Special thanks also to Julia Beaven from Wakefield Press who understood the necessity for this book and helped bring it to life.

Preface

Hardly a week goes by without some mention of the 'mentally ill' or 'mental illness' in the media. News coverage is given to funding for mental health services and the accompanying political manoeuvring, but also to the sensationalised accounts of escapes from 'mental institutions' or acts of violence committed by a person with a 'mental illness'.

In the advertising media the approach is different. A grindingly pleasant voice tells us that there is now 'help available' and that 'we' no longer need to suffer in silence. No doubt the intention of these ads is to in some way redress the stigma the news items may have created, but the 'niceness' of it all inevitably leaves me with vague distaste.

In the reality-TV world of chat shows, health programs and special news items, the portrayal of 'mental illness' mimics that of the medical world. We are shown the world of 'mental illness' from the outside looking in, much as a psychiatrist, doctor or psychologist might. A person with a 'mental illness' is depicted as a combination of cells, brain and behaviours . . . some or all of which have somehow gone askew. The latest advances are showcased: new medications, new behaviour modification strategies, new theories and new diagnoses. These, evidently, give cause for 'hope'.

If I go into a library or bookshop of a reasonable size I can find shelf upon shelf of books on 'mental illness': schizophrenia, depression, anxiety, bipolar disorder, multiple personality disorder, and so on. But once studied, it becomes clear that the majority of these books are written by professionals – psychiatrists, psychologists, therapists. The short biographies inside the front cover tell of people who have graduated with great distinction from this university or that and have a 25-year practice in a 'centre' somewhere. The book is endorsed by even more highly credentialed authorities on the subject. I imagine that these people live comfortably with their spouse and two children somewhere on the Australian or US coastline, far away from a life on the disability pension.

Apart from a select few autobiographies there is actually very little to be found on the 'mentally ill' themselves. It does not seem relevant to ask who these people are when they are not the subjects of case studies, medical interventions, sensationalism, superficiality or ignorance.

So who are the people we call 'mentally ill'? What do the words 'mental illness' mean to the people for whom they have been used?

The idea for a book that might answer these questions has been with me for a long time in one form or another. I considered a personal testimony, or a scholarly or academic study (perhaps with some personal experiences thrown in), that might provide a counterbalance to the experts. But in the end it became less important for me to add another neat answer or packaged solution to all those already available. And the pressing question remained: who are the *real* experts? I felt that only from the *inside* could all these questions truly be answered.

In 2004 I met a man called Patrick at a Lifeline counselling course. The first week we happened to sit next to each other, and then each week that followed we did the same. We started to chat. Patrick had a wonderful Irish brogue, a keen talent for storytelling, a deep insight and an uncommon humanity. As we spoke, the story of his life slowly unfolded and, as it did, so did my conviction that a wisdom such as his should be put down on paper. I also thought of the countless people I had spoken with over the years, and I thought of my own life. Here were rich lives, full lives and lives lived with questions. But here also were lives of suffering that at some time had been termed 'mental illness'.

I shared my idea for a book of interviews with Patrick. He was positive and encouraging. He understood its value and its necessity and saw my passion for the subject and the people. He agreed to be interviewed.

Once the book was a reality in my mind, I had to bring it to life. I thought through the logistics of such an enterprise. Uppermost in my mind was the fact that I would be interviewing people who may well be some of the most vulnerable in our society and who might share with me their deepest and often darkest moments. I understood that recounting such moments might prove intensely painful and challenging and could all too easily catapult people back into places they hoped they had left behind. From the beginning I was clear that I did not want the interview process to add to this pain. My interview style could not be brashly interrogative or confrontational in any way. I also felt it was necessary from the outset to make it clear that I had no agenda. I wasn't studying people. I merely wanted to relate as human being to human being, gently asking in my own mind, as I might of a friend, Who are you? What are your thoughts? What are your feelings? What is your life like? What do you think of when the words 'mental illness' are used? . . . and see what the outcome would be.

I also felt that if so desired, people *must* have the option of having all aspects of their privacy and confidentiality protected. I decided to draw up a contract which among other things, protected the rights of the interviewee, but also, in these times of litigation, protected me from any claims for damage.

The next step, of course, was finding people other than Patrick who might wish to be interviewed. I did not want to vet people. Not only did I feel that doing so might leave people with the sense that if I refused them they were not worthy, I also did not want to attract people who might necessarily share my points of view. I *did* however keep in mind that I wanted a group of people who had been given a range of diagnoses, and who were from a broad cross-section of society and age groups. I also felt it was important that these people were not currently experiencing an acute crisis, that they would value 'having a say', and were able to reflect with a degree of self-awareness on their lives.

I wrote a letter outlining the project. I listed my reasons for writing the book and made it clear that if desired all aspects of the interviewee's privacy and confidentiality would be protected. In the letter I also mentioned that for many years I had lived with the suffering that is termed 'mental illness'. On all counts this proved to be a point of meeting and understanding, even if not openly discussed.

Over the years that I carried out the interviews I occasionally sent this letter to various organisations asking if they knew of someone who might be interested in being interviewed. I also approached people and asked if they themselves, or someone they knew, might wish to be interviewed. Word of mouth, friend of a friend . . . slowly the list of interviewees grew. And as it did, I was astonished that the people who came to me did indeed represent a broad range of ages and diagnoses and were from a cross-section of society. The book grew as if by magic.

I found that those who wished to be interviewed generally did so for one or more of the following reasons:

- They felt a strong desire to educate people.
- They felt passionately about the stigmatisation, stereotyping and misconceptions surrounding 'mental illness'.
- They felt unheard, marginalised, infantilised or angered with regard to the treatment they had received.
- They felt that the story of their life might offer guidance, solace or encouragement to others who suffer.

Seventeen interviews are included in this book with people ranging in age from twenty to 74. It surprised me that only four people wished to have their identity protected. The remainder used their own names although not all wished to have their photos included. A few like Wayne, Linda and Glenda had a photo included from which they could not be readily identified.

The range of diagnoses includes schizophrenia, atypical schizophrenia, dissociative identity disorder, bipolar disorder, depression, generalised anxiety disorder, panic disorder, borderline personality disorder, phobias, obsessive compulsive disorder, and drug-induced psychosis.

The interviews cover an enormously broad range of topics including views on the nature of 'mental illness' and suffering, stigma, what it means to be a human being, opinions on the professional help available (including hospitalisation, therapy and electroconvulsive therapy (ECT)), suicide, self-harm, trauma, child abuse, cults, alcoholism, violence, crime, homelessness, AIDS, living with a physical disability, art, music, writing, nature, Aboriginality, spirituality, Christianity, the impact of war, the importance of relationships, illicit drug use, prescription drug use, side effects, mental health funding . . .

Once I had made phone or e-mail contact with a prospective interviewee we arranged to meet. I discussed the project briefly but did not allude in any way either to my own experience or points of view, or to those of other interviewees. I made it my practice to have no prearranged questions. I simply asked people to start at a point that was important for them and suggested that the interview might then proceed much like a conversation. The majority of people started with a description of their childhood, feeling that this was necessary for an understanding of their lives. (Some further notes on the language and technical details of the interviews are outlined in Appendix A.)

As an interview proceeded, I avoided bringing up

any topic that the interviewee themselves had not mentioned. I felt it was my job simply to listen, to be utterly present, to stay out of the way as much as possible and to only ask for clarification if I felt it was needed. Quite beyond my expectations, people shared with me their histories and memories, their innermost thoughts and feelings, their healing. They shared their lives and their dignity. Many told me there was much that they had talked about for the first time for the book. In the course of the interviews I came to feel privileged and deeply humbled.

All interviews were taped and the material written up afterwards. This was sent to the interviewee to read through. We then met again to discuss the material and add more to the interview. This process was repeated up to four times. As I had anticipated, the interviews were occasionally painful and exhausting but also, at times, filled with laughter and further discussions that were not included in the book. Many interviewees were astonished and deeply proud of the wisdom they read. A couple of people felt that the interview was the most important thing they had done with their lives. Many subsequently showed their interviews to family, friends, doctors or children in the hope that *now* they might be understood.

Not one person I interviewed needed to be persuaded of the value of the book. Indeed, it became apparent that many people were at a virtual bursting point in terms of their willingness and desire to talk. But, as many interviews allude to in some way, it was not just the desire to talk that was important, it was the act of being listened to. Sarah spoke after her interview about the significance of this. In many respects this paragraph also astutely sums up many of my reasons for writing this book.

The way you've presented the interview and the way you've been very open and accepting and accommodating of people's experiences and people's lived traumas is the opposite to our experiences in the everyday world. That's the reason this book is so important. Our voice, our need to reach out and be part of society is the reason this book needs to be written and the reason people need to hear our stories and listen to our experiences. Our lives are lived so closed. We try to hide our symptoms and present ourselves to society in a certain way. That only compounds our lives with a mental illness. The freedom and the ability to express ourselves is so important. People need to listen to our stories, listen to our points of view and have a different understanding of mental illness . . . I've often said that mental illness is a condition of society.

Some interviewees described how not being listened to in their lives and most particularly in their search for help, had led not only to frustration, hopelessness and re-traumatisation but also to violence, crime and attempted suicide. Many were only too clear about the enormous gulf between true listening and simply being heard. This is summed up by Joan:

I see a difference between listening and hearing. Some people might hear everything but not really *listen* to what you're saying, or to the feeling attached to what you're saying . . . if people listen, then you *know* they're listening by the fact that they understand where you're coming from.

and also Meg:

There are lots of people who hear you but they don't really *listen*. They don't listen to the intensity of what you're saying. They don't *know* it like you know it. They don't feel any true empathy. People are just polite and then it doesn't go any further.

Trevor adds:

> I think it's so important for professionals to *listen*. This is just as true of life as it is of psychiatry – *people need to learn to listen!* They would learn a lot more by just listening. Men are dreadfully bad at listening. They just tend to give solutions and that's not necessarily what people in crisis want.

My hope is that through this book, people living with 'mental illness' might truly be listened to by the general public and also by the professionals and politicians who hold the destiny of so many people in their hands. Simply by virtue of my capacity to *listen*, one interviewee suggested that I should be put in charge of all mental health funding, because then the money would be used where those who are suffering need it the most.

In this introduction I don't wish to pre-empt the content and the stories of the interviews, but I would like to point out that beyond listening there are many points of agreement that recur throughout the interviews. I hope that it will be these themes that most powerfully convey the humanity, the lives, the opinions, the desires, the difficulties, and the needs of people living with 'mental illness'. (Themes are summarised in Appendix B.)

Disclaimer

All opinions contained in the interviews are those of the interviewee alone and do not necessarily reflect the views of the author. At the request of some of the interviewees and paying heed to the fact that life and its circumstances can change quite dramatically, I add the stipulation that these interviews represent the interviewees' opinions at only *one* particular point in time.

No opinions are intended as professional advice, diagnosis, treatment or service. No opinions are intended to be a substitute for independent professional or therapeutic advice. No liability will be accepted if they are taken as such.

Marianne Broug, Adelaide

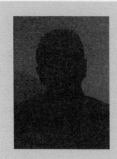

Wayne

Wayne is 55 years old. *'In describing myself I would rather call myself a father, a grandfather, a partner and a friend than someone who is Tasmanian, Aboriginal and living with a mental illness.'*

The very beginning

My father married my mother on the way to the Second World War, on the basis that should he die overseas, my mother would get the war widows' pension. But my father came back and I was born in Tasmania in the 1950s.

My mother has an Aboriginal background and so does my father. My mother does not acknowledge her Aboriginality and only on his deathbed did my father discuss his heritage.

My father was a travelling salesman for a company that sold beer, wine and spirits. He was away from home a lot. When my father was away travelling, my mother would put the OMO detergent packet up on the window to let all her friends know that the old man was out ('Old Man Out') and that they could come over to the house to drink beer. My father would not have let this happen.

From the time I was very young, alcohol played a big part in my life. My father and mother were both alcoholic. The little sample spirits bottles from my father's company were always lying around – crème de menthe and all that type of stuff. Even as a kid I used to get drunk. If a friend came over, I'd steal a couple of

1

bottles of beer and we'd open them with our teeth and drink them. I remember one time my stepmother had pissed in one of the bottles of beer . . . and I drank that by mistake!

My mother was a wanderer and would go walkabout with different men. She would come and go, come and go. Sometimes she would take us with her, sometimes she wouldn't. By the time I went to school at five, I had three younger siblings. Eventually my parents had fourteen children between them – all to various partners. I went to seven different primary schools.

And I was told I was a hyper-manic kid. I remember even on the first day of school, I threw a rock and it hit someone in the head. Although I put the onset of my mental illness much later in my life, I believe that if my childhood had been lived now, I would have been diagnosed with attention deficit disorder (ADD) or something similar. I've actually begun to wonder whether kids with ADD grow up to be adults with bipolar affective disorder.

Were you aware of your Aboriginality when you were young?

Only in my soul. It now plays a major part in my life, but as a child it did not. It is only on looking back that I recognise the importance of various incidents in my life.

When I was in school I made a pair of bookends in plaster depicting an Aboriginal man's head. I painted them black, varnished them and gave them to my grandmother. Perhaps I felt connected to Truganini or other Tasmanian Aboriginals! Do you know the Truganini story? She was the last of the Tasmanian Aboriginals. Her skeleton was kept in a museum. Remains of other people, including their heads, were taken overseas and then later returned. If I had looked at my feelings *then*, they would probably just have been compassion or something like that. Only in retrospect was it weird.

My grandfather, who was the lineage, did a couple of things that indicated his Aboriginality to me, although at the time I assumed that this was just what everyone did. My grandfather would take me fishing and cook the fish in the ground. He would also pick up seashells, boil them and then eat them. I also assumed that most people grew onions, took the frying pan with the extension lead down to the vegetable garden, heated it up and cooked the onions fresh.

As far as my mother goes, even though she didn't acknowledge her Aboriginality, she has lived her life with Aboriginal people. At one stage my mother's lover was Aboriginal. Later she went on to have a long-term relationship with a man whose mother was a traditional Aboriginal woman. My mother never wore shoes. She looks like a gin[1]. My mother always wanted a black baby. When I was young, my mother bought me a black baby doll to play with. To this day my mother and sisters live together in one house and they all barrack for the West Indies, they like watching Afro-American fighters, they have posters of Shaquille O'Neill[2] on the wall . . . black, black, black is all they think of . . .

And yet they do not identify at all with Aboriginal people?

No, no, no! It's weird . . . but my sister's children, my nieces, ask me, 'Uncle Wayne, Uncle Wayne, are we Aboriginal?' They ask *me*!

Why do they ask you?

---

1   Aboriginal woman

2   Afro-American basketball player

Because in early 1995 I developed my mental illness and that was as a direct result of going to Alice Springs and seeing the horrors with the Aboriginal people there. At that time there were a large number of rapes, there was violence, and I saw severe alcoholism and petrol sniffing. I remember as I was leaving Alice Springs by train, I saw people living in the creek bed and on the railway siding and it looked as if they had been left over from a war . . . I was terribly affected by everything I saw. After that my Aboriginality was in my brain.

Psychosis

At the time I went to Alice Springs, I lived in the country and was married with two children. While I was away my wife had decided to separate. The day I got back she said, 'Tomorrow I am leaving you.' And she left.

I was deeply distressed by this and as a result I went through four days of sleep deprivation during which I started to lose the plot . . . I started to develop a plan to save the Aboriginal people . . . and my plan was to ban petrol and replace it with marijuana! I decided to grow fields of marijuana! However the consequence of this was that the oil cartels from around the world would gang up to get rid of me.

Eventually I rang my wife who was staying with her parents in the city and I begged to see her. On my drive into the city, my psychosis really started to develop. I left my car at the city police station because I thought the Russian Mafia was following me. I caught a taxi from there to the house of my parents-in-law. I stayed there overnight and woke up early in the morning wanting a priest . . . wanting sanctuary, wanting asylum, wanting a safe place . . . I thought people in cars with guns were surrounding the house.

My father-in-law is a pistol shooter and so I woke him up saying, 'Get your guns. Get your guns they're surrounding us!' Then I jumped the back fence and thought I was going to a monastery not far away. Instead I went to a nearby Catholic residential care facility for the elderly that was run by nuns. It was a nursing home with security buttons and stuff.

I went into this place, and there was a twenty-foot statue of Jesus! I thought I was at the monastery. I pressed a button and a voice asked, 'What can we do to help you?' I said, 'I want to see a priest.' I held what I thought was my driver's licence up to a security camera, but it wasn't . . . it was my firearms licence! The nuns or hospital staff rang the police. The staff then let me in and made me a cup of tea while we waited for the police. Two police came in, a man and a woman. They took me back to my father-in-law's place and asked my wife what they should do. She said, 'Take him to S . . .' I was back in their car, quite happy . . .

Were you aware that S . . . was a psychiatric hospital?

No! Of course not! I was happy to be with the police. I must have been completely disoriented. I waltzed into S . . . 'dah da dah da dah' . . . and had no idea of mental illness whatsoever, even though I'd witnessed some of the de-institutionalisation and met people living with mental illness. In the early '90s we had owned a deli and lived in the house behind. Nearby were the boarding houses where they put the people from the local psychiatric hospital . . . with whom I got on *wonderfully* well, by the way . . . they were eccentric, they were characters, they'd come in of a night . . .

Anyway I reached out my hand to say goodbye to the police and the male police officer shook my hand.

I reached for that of the female officer and she went for her gun! Then it hit me. Bang! I realised I was in hospital. So then I asked for an *Aboriginal psychiatrist*! That was probably my first mistake.

What was their reaction?

Well coincidentally, all the psychiatrists *were* black! They were from other cultures . . . not Aboriginal of course . . . but my psychiatrist *was* black . . . and then after that I forget what happened . . . blank . . . I was zombied . . . I was medicated. I think they probably just wanted to shut me up. 'Where am I? Who am I? Count backwards in sevens.' I don't remember anything until they transferred my care to the local hospital.

The local hospital also gave me a good dose of pills. I was given a female psychiatrist who was also from another country . . . also black. She came with the medication and I asked, 'What happens when I take all this medication?' and she said, 'Well if you ask questions like that you'll only get more!' That's all I remember . . . I have since spoken to people I was in hospital with and I may well have been non-compliant.

Time moved on . . . days went by . . . I slept . . . and then slept some more . . . and then after a while I started to get the hang of what was going on . . . Then one day one of the staff came by and asked, 'Do you want to go to church, Wayne?' I was taken to church with some other guy from the hospital who thought he was the son of the wrestler Hulk Hogan and was waiting for the Hale Bop Comet to come by so he could jump on its tail and go back home. So off we went to church. They sat us in a small room and started speaking in tongues to try to de-possess us! *I ran out of that church and back to hospital!* Can you *believe* that?

They tried to exorcise you?

Yes. Lay hands. Speak in tongues! . . . These guys had come into the hospital in their ties and suits, all very nice . . .

Did the hospital know what they intended?

No. No. My daughter was also going to church at the time and she was given a 47-day prayer program for the mentally ill . . . because in the eyes of some churches mental illness is seen as demonic possession. She had to pray for my soul, night after night after night!

Anyway, I went back to hospital and I immediately started to play the game, because to me, God is good not bad. And those guys were *bad*! I knew I had to get out of hospital and I rapidly became compliant. For instance, I instigated 'Rules for Art' – I recycled all the medication containers to save on paint. I did a big chart with all the rules written down and fancy pictures around the edges – 'Don't Waste the Paint', 'Wash your Brushes' . . . I was probably quite grandiose but I was playing their game . . . they got me stabilised and normalised and tranquillised and counting backwards . . . and I was discharged.

Before I'd gone to Alice Springs I had planned a holiday with my wife and kids and I still wanted to do that. And so we went on holiday. But while we were away, my wife and kids said, 'That's it, we can't stay with you any more!' I was mad *as*!

How were you mad?

I had stopped taking the medication and had become hyper-manic . . . I spent money, I stayed awake, I watched videos, I wanted to visit old friends . . . we didn't have a very good time, but all the same, when we returned home my wife and I reconciled.

By mid '96 I was reasonably unpsychotic. I was on lithium and an anti-psychotic/tranquiliser and my thoughts were coming together . . . I was okay except for the side effects. I was sleeping twenty hours a day and putting on massive amounts of weight. But I did work in an adult retreat on the weekends. The lady who ran it was a nurse and she was very understanding and good to me. Apart from this I had no other life – no social life. I *did* begin to study Community Services, and eventually started doing paramedical-aide work with the frail aged, under the instruction of a physiotherapist.

In 1997 my wife had a car accident. It wasn't serious, but I was certain that I had made it happen. I was sure that it was my fault and that I had somehow wanted her dead. Then one day when I was wheeling the washing basket out to the clothesline, the basket suddenly became my wife in a wheelchair. I vomited and my brain exploded . . . another bout of psychosis.

It was also around this time that the issue of my sexuality came up. I was not fulfilling my role as a husband. I went to the doctor complaining of my loss of libido. I felt asexual. It was not an issue for my wife, but I felt that I had lost a part of me. As I remember saying to my son, 'Where is the man part? Where has it gone?' I saw my wife as some sort of 'black thing'; it was as though there was darkness around her. If I came into the house it was as though it had darkness in it.

I had assumed that my sexuality had been altered by mental illness and by medication. I remember sitting around once with a few guys and we were whingeing because of the lack of intimacy in our lives, blaming it on our lack of desire, our unattractiveness because of the medication and whatever else we could find to blame. But that was a delusion I was living with at the time. On reflection, I realised that it went a lot further back . . .

Further back . . .

When I was nine and in grade three I had a testicular hernia. Even though I had an operation to correct it, I spent most of my teenage years believing I could never have children; I assumed I was impotent. I realise that sexuality is more than the act of sex, but in my mind I assumed I was sterile. (Certainly I later disproved all this when at the age of seventeen I had a daughter!)

How had the testicular hernia come about?

In my mind, I was getting some wood off a wood-pile and the wood fell down and crushed me. I hurt my knees and there was a lump in my stomach . . . I remember that Mum ran a bath and while I was in the bath she pushed the lump and I vomited into the bath. I remember the doctor coming and then my mother taking me to hospital. I was in hospital for a month and I think I was off school for nine. I had two operations.

And this is my first memory of hallucinations . . . this may or may not be true . . . perhaps they gave me a pre-med and it was a drug-induced psychosis . . . I feel that there were nuns there with candles wheeling me around . . . During the operation angels with candles looked down from an observatory . . . and I also saw Jesus hovering there with his arms outstretched . . . but it may just have been a big statue. I don't know. But that was the last time I saw my mum for a fair while. She never visited me in hospital.

Why?

In retrospect my sister has negated the story of the woodpile falling on me. I don't want to hear these stories.

What is your sister saying?

If I can be explicit? . . . I've got a hole in my arm that I always thought came from swinging on a tyre in the barn. My loving sister was pushing me and I accidentally fell onto a pitchfork. However, when I was recounting the episode to my sister in '97 she said, 'I speared you. I wanted to kill you' . . . And it was then that we got onto the story of how my testicular hernia had come about . . . she says that I was tied to the clothesline and bashed with a lump of wood . . .

Was your childhood a violent one?

My parents were violent to one another. My mother would break a beer bottle over my father's head. My father would hold my mother back with a broom. And there was, 'Wait till your father gets home'. And the jug cord. And the belt and all that. But it wasn't traumatic enough to be embedded. *Or* I've replaced these incidents with accidents . . . at one stage my arm was broken . . . I said I had done it 'playing basketball', even though I'd never played basketball in my life. I don't know what happened to my arm.

But after the incident with the testicular hernia and the subsequent hospitalisation, I went to live with my paternal grandparents, and did so until they died. During my teenage years I went to *one* high school. When I married at eighteen we lived with my grandparents and had a wonderful life. My wife and I both had jobs, cars and boats.

My grandparents loved me dearly, more than their own son (my father). When they died they left *me* their estate, and not my father. He contested the will, but he was unsuccessful. My father and I did not speak again for over twenty years. But I lost the plot after they died. I started drinking every day, drinking when I woke up, drinking when I went to sleep. I was spending as much money in hotels as I was earning. Eventually it got too much for my wife and we separated.

In 1972 I sold the house that I had inherited to a returned Vietnam veteran I had met in a hotel. The house was fully furnished, had food in the fridge, a lawn mower, everything . . . I left Tasmania with the money under the mat in the car. Looking back this episode seems a *very* appropriate description of mental illness . . . although undiagnosed and untreated.

For two years I drove around Australia towing a covered trailer with a few treasured possessions from my grandmother and some clothes. I met Aboriginal people up in Arnhem Land and in the Western Desert, and all I felt was empathy. I thought, 'This is where I want to be'. I met Aboriginal people who had not seen a white person. But I had no concept of Aboriginality then.

After travelling for two years I got a job, got married again and settled down. When my daughter was born I didn't want to do shift work any more, so I started my own property maintenance business. We had another child, a son, and we bought that deli I mentioned earlier. We built it up and up . . . and in 1991 we sold it and moved to the country . . . And then '95 happened . . .

'What are ya?'

Since then I've been diagnosed with bipolar schizo-affective disorder. They gave me a booklet on bipolar and a booklet on schizophrenia and asked me which one I wanted to be. I was medicated with both mood stabilisers and anti-psychotics. I remember going to a mental health resource centre and I wasn't sure whether I wanted to be with the schizophrenia people down-stairs or with the mood disorders mob upstairs. The mood disorders mob was a bit derogatory about those downstairs. I had always been more comfortable with the underclass and so preferred the downstairs schizophrenia people to the moody bastards upstairs!

But if someone asks, 'What are ya?' I would not say I have schizophrenia. I would say 'I have been diagnosed, treated, hospitalised and medicated with bipolar' . . . probably because I too stigmatise against people with schizophrenia! It's the labelling thing! I don't want to be one of them! . . . even if I am! Imagine that . . . a Tasmanian Aboriginal with schizophrenia!

But I do know that I see things and hear things . . . I remember once in *South Park* they had a nurse with a conjoined foetus on her shoulder . . . I hallucinated that for so long that my psychiatrist just about shook me, 'Don't go there, Wayne! Don't go there!' I was driving along in the car thinking that I had a conjoined foetus on my shoulder.

And today I had a wonderful vision . . . I was looking through glass at the front of a hotel and it turned into a waterfall. The only reason I knew it wasn't real was that I said to the guy I was with, 'Hey look at that waterfall!' He said to me, 'There's no waterfall there, Wayne.' I looked back and there was no waterfall.

Taking into account your life overall, what is your view on the nature of mental illness?

My view is that you're born with it and that it needs a trigger, and the depth of the perception of what that trigger is . . .

I feel my greatest trauma was being separated from my mother's breast to go to school. My mother seems to think that I wanted the breast even when I came home from school. But of course by then my next three siblings were having a go at it. It's a big big joke between us. Even now she says to me, 'You want the titty bottle, Wayne?' I can remember the smell of my mother . . . the menstrual smell of my mother . . . I can remember . . .

You feel that being separated from your mother's breast was a trauma that affected the development of your mental illness?

Yep. Yep. I had no contact with my mother from the time of the hospitalisation until I had my daughter at seventeen. It was as though not only my mother's breast went, but my *whole* mother went as well. I relate the loss of my mother to the breast thing, because then I can trivialise it a bit more. Rather than saying, 'My mother left me' I can say, 'I was taken off the breast at five!' . . . it can be a bit of joke because other people were taken off the breast at the age of one and don't remember a thing about it.

A psychiatrist

I am very very happy with the way my psychiatrist operates. My relationship with him is very important to me. I can't speak of him too highly. I've spoken to the professor who taught my psychiatrist and he said that my psychiatrist could not be taught anything and that everything he knows he taught himself.

Is the way he works different to other psychiatrists?

Yes. Very different.

I first went to see him for my son. He said, 'Your son is okay. It's *you* that I want to see.' At my first appointment, I asked him, 'What model are we going to work on here?' I suppose I was trying to be grandiose or a smart-arse. And he said to me, 'We'll talk about whatever you want to talk about, whenever you want to talk about it.'

I came to see him medicated. One of the medications was a particular anti-psychotic/tranquiliser that no one in their right mind would ever take again. *Ever!* One of the side effects of the medication was that my vision had become impaired. He spoke about the inappropriate levels of medication that I had been given. Because my condition was mild and because I had '*insight*' he was happy that once the lithium worked I could stop all other medications. He then helped me through the medication reduction. He told me that if I decided to take myself off lithium and as a result lost the plot then that was *my* choice. He also said that if I wanted medication I would have to get it from my GP. He didn't want me coming to him to get medication.

What were his reasons for not prescribing medication?

I'm not sure whether it was to avoid litigation or whether he genuinely felt that it was not his job to be medicating people and forcing them to be on a medication regime for the rest of their lives. He was there to talk. If I have an issue that I feel is worth talking about then he will talk about it. I go to him with whatever issues are current in my life and he will generally have a view on those topics. The fact that what we talk about is of immediate relevance to my life is very important. Talking has helped me *so much more* than medication. Medication put me to bed, reduced my motivation and increased my weight. He is a confidante who I can speak to about things, without having them negated.

Could you go into a little more detail about the ways in which talking has helped you?

When I first went on the disability support pension, I saw that as bringing three negatives into my life: disability, support and pension. My psychiatrist suggested that rather than looking at it negatively, I look at it as my government payment or a way of getting my taxes back. I found that very helpful.

He also encouraged me to insist on payment for my participation in consultations with the mental health service. In retrospect I often see that people *do* undervalue themselves. He helped me to lift my self-esteem by providing an opportunity for me to realise that I wasn't worthless and hopeless.

And then I might tell him stories . . . about my father and Christmas for instance. His father was born on Christmas Day and so was mine, and so we'd talk about how each of them had coped with sharing their birthday with Jesus. My father would ignore birthdays. So then he'd say, 'Your father is an arsehole!' . . .

I'd come in and say, 'My wife told me that people like me shouldn't be allowed to breed.' And then he'd say, 'Fuck, did she say that?' He actually advised me to get out of my marriage. Whether that's an ethical thing to do or not, I don't know, but afterwards he said he had seen so many people get out of destructive relationships and start a new life. And I was able to do that. In retrospect it *was* the best move I could have made. Because of my illness I had been pretty well de-powered in my marriage, and there was no way in the world that my wife was going to relinquish any of her power and control. I could have no input into anything, whether it was the kids, buying a computer, selling a house . . . even if I suggested something as trivial as going on a picnic it would never happen. I didn't even have any choice on clothing or friends.

A major thing he also gave me was a knowledge of what to do around my sensitivity. Apparently I am over-sensitive and there's no book on such things, no medication . . .

In what way are you sensitive?

Personal sensitivities. I don't want to be called 'little' or 'small' for instance. He taught me how to block out comments like that. He told me to pretend that I was a knight in shining armour and that nothing could penetrate.

I was also *overly* sensitive to international incidents. I was extremely paranoid that my kids were going to get shot at school because of the school shootings in the US. The starving children in Africa affected me greatly. I'd talk about it so much that one day my daughter said to me, 'I hate those bloody starving kids in Africa!' He reduced my anxiety by telling me that these are worldwide issues and that I could move my focus onto my own life. He told me that the likelihood of these things happening in my backyard was very remote.

He is also available to me outside of appointment times. When my father died last November (on Melbourne Cup day) my partner rang my psychiatrist because I was not reacting. He told my partner that he would ring me back in one hour's time. And he did. I also remember going to a funeral at which I was to give the eulogy. I rang him just before it started, to tell him that I was anxious and I was about to take some tranquillisers. He said, 'It's only twenty minutes to go, Wayne, what's the point? You'll be right.' And I was. I have his mobile number, his work number and his home number.

Has his approach been a major part of taking you forward in your life?

There were probably three things that happened in tandem that have got me where I am. Had I not had the psychiatrist and had continued blindly accepting medication from my wife, I may well still have been in that homebound situation. I also got involved with a psychosocial rehabilitation centre in a nearby town. It's a non-government organisation where people with mental illness can go. It is a safe supportive zone where people recovering from mental illness are *respected*! They aren't treated differently from anyone else and are allowed to get on with their recovery at their own pace. I've been involved with that group for seven years. And the third thing is my current partner. We've been together almost six years. She gives me acceptance and understanding. She accepts me as I am. She respects my choices in life and also my ability to choose what clothes I want to wear, what I want to do with my hair, where we want to go, the friends we want to have . . . Freedom. I have freedom now that I did not have.

Aboriginality

At the beginning of the interview you mentioned that your Aboriginality now plays a major part in your life. How did that come about?

When I got out of hospital and a year or two went by, I was asked to be a mental health advocate on an Aboriginal health forum. I wasn't asked as an Aboriginal person, but rather as someone who could talk mental health issues with the forum. I went along and slowly started meeting Aboriginal people, particularly in the area where I live.

As life went on, a position on that forum for a community representative became vacant, and so I went along and spoke to in excess of twenty Aboriginal people, saying to them, 'I'm here, happy to take your views to the regional service as an Aboriginal person. This is my history, I was born in Tasmania . . .' I was never asked to supply DNA or anything. I was just accepted.

So then I began to do community consultations around the Aboriginal Primary Health Care Access Project. We have funding from the unused Medibank monies. Medibank was not accessed by Aboriginal people, so the pool of money that remained is currently being put back into Aboriginal health at $170 per head per annum. We have 1000 of those heads, so we have $170,000 to access primary health care. I've been involved in community consultations with Aboriginal people in our zone: What do you want? Where do you want to access primary health care? Would you access a mainstream GP?

So these questions are to do with health per se and not just mental health.

It is funded through health, but the social determinates of health are art, education, justice and housing. Mental health was the vehicle that got me into Aboriginal health. The mental health component of Aboriginal health got thrown out, shredded and put in a bin because Aboriginal people would prefer not to look at it as mental 'illness' (as it was then) but rather as an issue of social and emotional well-being. Should it be an incident of voices coming from the ancestors after death, it's not schizophrenia, it's a social and emotional issue that traditional healers or counselling with an elder could help the person to get through. Rather than depression we'd be speaking of grief and loss. It's a different kettle of fish.

Do people have access to traditional healing?

No. Where we come from there is no concept of traditional healing and as such there are no traditional healers. The Aboriginal people have been mainstreamed, medically, religiously and societally. The people have had traditional models taken away from them and replaced by Christianity. In the local Aboriginal community for instance, the elders said, 'We will give up our language, we will give up our culture and we will embrace Catholicism. We won't speak like *that* any more, we won't act like *that* any more and we won't have any of those rituals.' It has been lost.

After consulting with the community what did you find that the Aboriginal people in your region wanted?

As a result of community consultation, we found out that they wanted a space or place that could be used as a meeting place or drop-in centre. They wanted a place where they could go. And it's also important to know what Aboriginal people *don't* want: they don't want to visit an institution, whether a hospital, school or gaol. The other day we were talking about getting some people to do a course in Senior First Aid. People were happy to do it, but only in their own town. They didn't want to travel. That comfort-zone stuff is very important for Aboriginal people.

We have now established a place like that in our town called 'The Meeting Place'. We've contracted a GP to come in once a week. An art group also meets there once a week. The funding for the rent of the building comes from the Aboriginal health forum's access to the unused Medibank money. The regional health service has funded the art space program, the computers, furniture, blinds, barbecue etc.

By setting up such a meeting place are you then able to address the issues of 'social and emotional well-being'?

Yes. Other than the GP and the art classes, it's a place where people can just drop in and have a yarn. Aboriginal people are taking ownership of it and the broader community has also accepted it. A couple of non-indigenous people have even asked if they can join the art group.

We've also had barbecues for which the hospital has supplied the meat. Probably every three months or so we have what we call a 'Healthy Day'. The Health Service comes along and might bring a physiotherapist, a diabetes educator or an asthma educator. We get the kids out of the schools, and have a family fun day type of thing with face painting, jazz-ercise and then a talk on asthma or diabetes or whatever. Next year we're planning to have these days at different places – perhaps at the golf course, or at the jetty, and then have fishing as one of the activities, or shell collecting, or playing golf.

What impact did it have on you personally when you started to speak as an Aboriginal person?

If an eagle swoops down in front of me and picks up a mouse, that's something I would look at. If there were two galahs sitting on a fence or a dead magpie on the road, all those things would have meant something to me, well and truly before all this. What does it mean if I see a bird flying through a sun shower? A sun shower is a mixture of good and bad. It's a rare occurrence. It might mean to increase my awareness or it might be an indication to take care. I draw more on signs and symbols, without seeing it as a problem any more.

Did you see it as a problem?

It was probably '97 before I started seeing a psychiatrist regularly and it wasn't even an issue I would bring up with him. It was something that I kept down. I had a feeling that if I had spoken to people about it then, it would have been seen as something that was part of my mental illness. That was certainly the feeling I was getting from my wife at the time: 'These are symptoms of your mental illness, Wayne. Delusion.' A lot of people even thought that my desire to go to the desert and be with Aboriginal people was a psychosis: 'Wayne's mad!'

So yeah, I felt weird. If I saw a galah stuck in a fence I would feel compelled to free it. If I saw a bird struggling in the snow, I would put it in the glove box to allow it to warm up. These are now symbolic to me of life and death, but in the old days I wouldn't have been able to say that. It would have been further proof that I was mad.

Today I saw a beautiful wedge-tailed eagle and I saw kites swooping down on the mice because they're ploughing the paddocks . . . now there's no abnormality associated with it. There's no madness in it now. I know people have totem animals and people have skin names. I feel freer now . . . but I also feel more able to listen and to talk and to accept. In the past I would have been more dismissive of people who were different. In the past I would have been anti-Asian, a redneck . . . I believed that trees were there to be cut down . . .

I also feel a strong connection to the land now. I feel a very strong connection to the land I own and I have an enormous respect for the Country whose land I am living on. I am happy to go along with their rights, their views on skeletal remains or whatever. When I go to the city, I am aware whose land I am on. I know where the meeting places were. It's the same in the Territory and on the Islands.

Do you feel that this awareness was something that was carried through in you, without any conscious direction?

Oh yeah! I feel that there *is* ancestral DNA. I believe it to be a case of ancestral DNA when the ancestors visit people at times of grief, loss or death. However, because there is no intellectual knowledge of such things, it becomes a frightening occurrence for them. On top of that they might be told that such visitations are a symptom of schizophrenia and that only compounds the problem. Then people resort to alcohol and other drugs . . . and then it's 'tie a rope around my neck and jump out of a tree'. Without the impact of a traditional healer and without any of the talking therapies, it might mean many years of suffering for those people.

The future?

The fact that my two daughters have had children has, in my mind, completed my purpose on this planet. I had heart surgery two years ago, and if I had died then, I would not have lived to see my grandchildren. I'm more at ease with everything – my Aboriginality, my children. One of the criteria for having the wisdom of an elder is to have grandchildren and now I feel I get that respect. It is also a common bond to talk about your children and grandchildren.

I feel I still have twenty years left and I've got short-term, medium-term and long-term goals. By the time I'm 60 I will have gone with my partner on three-month trips to Queensland, Northern Territory and Western Australia. There are so many places I would like to revisit, so many things I would like to show to my partner . . . Alice Springs, Broome, Kakadu . . . the colours, the creek beds, the sunrises and sunsets, sleeping in swags, the *stars* . . . and Aboriginal people. We've had some time on Palm Island and in our community and my partner has been accepted into the Aboriginal zone of life. There's no reason why that can't continue in other places.

I intend to continue doing what I'm doing with the Aboriginal health forum and I still have many goals with regard to my work in the community. For instance, there's an island nearby that in the future will be used for Aboriginal alcohol and drug rehabilitation. For the last three or four years it has been my desire to be involved with that. Yesterday I completed my Diploma in Community Services so I'm hoping that will get me in there, at the very least to assist in setting up programs and accessing funding.

As far as my mental illness goes, I don't want to die of depression any more. I don't even have those thoughts. My moods are generally more elevated. My verbosity, my level of activity and the fact that I stay awake are only a problem for other people. But I have insight. I accept that I have a mental illness and I respond really well when people tell me that I'm being inappropriate in my actions or speech. I know I can get excited and overspeak people, but when someone says something I am able to change. 'You've given 110 per cent, Wayne, but now it's time for you to take a little break!'

As far as my hallucinations go, they're not really a problem. I never hallucinate anything demonic. The only scary thing was the conjoined foetus. There's an old church across the road from where we live, and when we first moved in I told my partner that I could often see Jesus in the tree next to it. But I don't see mushrooms as big as houses on the road when I'm driving or anything like that. When I was really unwell I checked my car before I got into it in case someone was in there. I sometimes thought I was bugged and if a plane flew overhead I thought I was being followed. Sometimes I also thought

I was getting messages from the news when I listened to the radio. But I don't do these things any more. When I was anxious I used to hear a phone ringing and occasionally I still get that. Sometimes I'll ask my partner, 'Is that my phone ringing?' She'll just say, 'I can't hear it.'

I don't look on my mental illness as being a negative thing in my life. Without it I would not have had the life I've had. I know my life has been enormously up and down, but the fact is, when you pull that curvy line into a straight line then it's one hell of a lot longer than many others I know! I think I've done a hell of a lot with my life . . . from the very beginning I've done a hell of a lot!

Leah

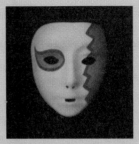

Leah is 20 years old. *'I wanted a photo of a mask here, because I walk around in society and nobody knows what I've been through. It's like I'm walking around with a mask on because nobody can see what's happened on the inside. Nobody understands the stresses I've been under. If they look at me they'll think I'm just a normal person.'*

Going into the psychosis hit me like a truck. I had a few warning signs, but it was more like I flipped out because I was on drugs. I was on speed, dope and depression tablets and it all just built up and exploded.

How long had you been taking the speed and the dope?

About four months.

How did you get into drugs?

My boyfriend. He gave me the drugs. When you're living and hanging around with someone who's doing it, you get dragged down into their world.

What was it like to take the speed and dope?

The dope was relaxing and when I took the speed I could do things I normally couldn't do. Things I wouldn't have had the patience for.

Like what?

I drew a picture of a bar scene when I was on speed. It took me twelve hours to do. I was just sitting there figuring out what would be in a bar scene. My brain was just *working* . . . a piano, a singer, a guy going on a date, glasses, a toilet, tables . . . I was thinking, 'And what else would go in there?' The wall isn't just a wall, it's a *curved*

wall. The door isn't just a door, it's tiled! It felt good . . .
and I just kept doing it.

And what about the antidepressants? Had they been prescribed for you?

Yeah. My boyfriend took me to the doctor.

Why did he take you to the doctor?

Because I'd started to cut myself. I was cutting my wrists. Making scratches and marks. For attention . . .

Were you doing anything else?

I put a bag over my head to suffocate myself when I went to sleep . . . I'd also gone into a deep depression. I was crying all the time and I didn't know why. I was also saying stupid things.

Like what?

Just little things. I went up to this boy I'd known a long time called Luke and tried to start a relationship even though he was already in one. I went around believing we already had a relationship.

When you put the plastic bag over your head, did you want to kill yourself?

I didn't just want to kill myself . . . I wanted to be sick enough so that someone would notice what was happening inside . . . I wanted to get attention from my boyfriend.

Did you want someone to listen to you?

Yeah. I was screaming inside but no one was listening . . . and it was just coming out as hurting myself. I was trying to make someone listen to my screams of needing help.

What did it feel like when you weren't listened to?

It kicks you in the guts, especially when you're going through so many traumas at the same time. I wanted someone I cared about to say, 'I care about you too.' I wanted a shoulder to cry on.

What had you been going through around this time?

My uncle, who I was very close to, had died. When I was a young girl I had been sexually molested. The person who molested me was at my uncle's funeral and he apologised to me. And that kind of set me to thinking about it a lot . . . it put a face to the person who had done it. That stressed me out a bit.

Had you remembered what had happened before he apologised?

Yeah. Part of it. But it brought things up again. When things like molestation happen, you always think you've done something wrong. You feel guilty. I wanted my boyfriend to hear about it. He wasn't listening very well.

So what happened when you went to the doctor?

I told him what I was going through and he prescribed me antidepressants and sent me home. But then I misused them. I started taking more than I should to make myself feel better. I took three every now and again when I felt bad. That's what my boyfriend was doing. He was taking them as well.

He was taking yours?

Yeah.

Did they help you to feel better?

They did. They made me feel happier. But so did the speed and the dope.

Then one day I rang my friends because I wanted them to come over to help me break up with my boyfriend because things weren't working out between us. I hadn't eaten for a couple of days because I was on drugs and everything. I was a mess. One moment I was crying and the next moment I was happy as Larry. Then I would start crying again and being all weird. I also felt really angry from time to time even when I had no reason to be angry. I was over-emotional. I think that at that point I may already have been under the psychosis.

Anyway I asked my friends to take my boyfriend for a drive and while they were out I took an overdose. I took eight antidepressants all at once to try to kill myself even though I knew it wasn't enough. I gulped them down as my friends were coming back in the door. They looked at the empty packet and then looked around the house to see if I might have hidden them somewhere to get attention. They didn't find anything. They told me it was a stupid thing to do. They said afterwards that they'd noticed I was acting strange. They also said afterwards that they felt really guilty that they hadn't told my parents what I had done.

I asked my friends to leave and then I just got higher and higher. The pills sent me on this real high. Because I felt better, I got back together with my boyfriend for about five hours. We got a bag of dope and I calmed down. Then later I rang up another friend and told him I was too scared to break up with my boyfriend because last time he had broken the remote control and the phone.

After that I can't really remember much . . . it all blurs together . . . I was flipping around . . . I wasn't sleeping . . . I wasn't feeling tired at all even though I had stayed up for days . . .

At one stage I was at my parents' house and I kept looking for Luke. I thought he was in the shed. I kept going out to the shed and knocking on the door, trying to get in, saying, 'I know he's in there'. During this time I was also trying to change myself for Luke. I thought I would become a piano teacher to impress him and so I sat at the piano for about twelve hours, practising hard. Later I was calling out for help because I thought that Dad was trying to hurt me when I was really trying to hurt him. He had locked all the doors to keep me safe in the house, but I smashed a window and tried to crawl out. I was screaming out that I needed help when I didn't need help. Eventually they had to call the ambulance. The ambulance and the police came and they took me to the psychiatric ward at the local hospital.

I was walking around the ward telling everyone I had schizophrenia when I didn't. I was literally out of my mind. I lost control of my bearings. It felt like I had no control over what I said even though I knew exactly what I was saying when I was saying it. I also thought I was psychic.

You thought you could read other people's minds?

No they could read mine but I couldn't read theirs because I was a deaf psychic. I was walking around yelling stuff. I thought I was just on my own in the world. I thought my father and brother had died because the police had shot them. When my dad came to visit me in hospital I actually thought he wasn't real. I thought I was seeing things. I also thought one of the symptoms of the speed was that I would die so that I could get this special serum to fix myself. I also thought Luke was in the hospital with me. I thought he was just hiding.

At first the hospital didn't really know what I had. At first it was 'drug-induced psychosis' then it was changed to 'schizophrenia' and then it was back to 'drug-induced psychosis' and then it was 'schizophrenia form disorder'. I felt a bit confused and angry that they didn't know what was wrong with me, particularly when they said I was schizophrenic. I had been walking around the ward saying I was schizophrenic but I knew I wasn't. And anyway, someone as sick as I was, wouldn't have been able to self-diagnose. I don't think they knew what they were talking about.

What is schizophrenia form disorder?

It's schizophrenia but you haven't had it for over six months. It looks like it is, but they can't say it is just yet.

Do *you* see the whole episode as drug induced?

It's so hard to know where the drugs stopped and the psychosis started. I believe I wouldn't have had the psychosis if I hadn't been on drugs.

What was your time in hospital like?

At first, when I was badly in the psychosis, it went really quickly. But then I was transferred to the major psychiatric hospital because I kept going into people's rooms, invading privacy and taking stuff. I didn't realise I was doing it. I'd just look at something I was holding in my hand and wonder, 'Where did I get this from?'

One incident I thought was really funny . . . when they were getting me ready to go to the psychiatric hospital, they stabbed me in the butt with a sedative. I didn't react to it, so they stabbed me in the butt with another one and I stood up and said, 'Is anything supposed to be happening yet?' They were expecting me to go, 'Phew!' and collapse but nothing happened. Eventually the ambulance came to take me away and I wasn't sedated at all. But I would never go to that psychiatric hospital again if I could help it.

Why?

Because it's scary. It's awful. There were lots of people in there with me. I didn't feel safe at all. It felt like gaol. Even the meals were like gaol.

So the psychiatric ward at the local hospital hadn't been scary?

No, it wasn't scary.

What was the difference between the two?

The major psychiatric hospital was closed in by a fence. And it was a closed ward. People there were *crazy* crazy and not just stressed-out crazy. I didn't get as much privacy. A lot of people in the local hospital just had depression and there weren't many people going through what I was going through. It felt safe there and my mum and dad could come and visit me there whenever they wanted. At the major psychiatric hospital I had to be let out into a certain room to visit with them.

Was there a difference in the way you were treated?

At the local hospital I was just treated like a sick person. At the psychiatric hospital there were a few mean people, but there were also a few nice ones. The mean ones were rough with me when I did things wrong. They put me in a solitary room when I was acting up. I've got Crohn's Disease and when you need to go to the toilet, you *need* to go to the toilet. They locked me in the solitary room and I was banging on the door saying, 'I need to go to the toilet! I need to go to the toilet!' . . . but they couldn't hear me. I wasn't very comfortable after that, put it that way! It wasn't very nice.

Did they know you have Crohn's Disease?

I don't know.

Did you see psychiatrists while you were in there?

Yeah I did. They just prescribed medication. They just asked me how I was feeling and whether I was getting better. I don't really know what they were trying to do. They were just medicating me.

Did you talk with anyone about the fact that you had been taking speed and dope and that you were cutting yourself?

No. They didn't really ask. I'm more of a you–ask–the–

questions-and-then-I'll-answer-them type of person. If you don't ask the question then I won't tell you.

So people have to ask the right questions?

Nobody asked the right questions. If they had asked, 'Are you still hallucinating butterflies?' I would have said 'yes'. I thought butterflies were a sign from God. I started looking for things related to butterflies ... room 21 in the hospital had a butterfly on the door and I kept going in there. The butterflies were meant to lead me to the right places.

What were the wrong questions?

'Do you hear voices?' I never heard voices. They kept saying that I heard voices, but I told them that I never heard them. They never got that. That's why they were saying I was schizophrenic ... because they thought I was hearing voices. They didn't believe it when I said that I wasn't hearing voices.

At first when I wanted to learn about psychosis I read a lot about it. I researched it myself. I researched the different forms it can take and realised I could have had any one of them. I could have had a drug-induced psychosis. I could have had another one because I had a fixation and mistaken belief that I was going out with Luke. There is a psychosis brought on by stress. There is one brought on by bipolar. I could have had a whole lot of things. But I never really thought I had schizophrenia because the main thing is hearing voices. I wanted a correct diagnosis.

Eventually they transferred me back to the open ward at the local hospital because I was getting better. I was on an anti-psychotic and a mood stabiliser. It took me about another two weeks to get fully better ... well I wasn't actually fully better ... a person in there convinced me that it would be better if I didn't mention to anyone that I still thought I was psychic. So I went in to the doctor and said 'Oh yeah, I don't think I'm psychic any more' and they let me go. I was still in the psychosis when I left hospital and then I got worse and worse. I went in again three weeks later. I still felt psychic. I still felt that I was special. I thought I could see ghosts and stuff like that. My mum found me at four o'clock in the morning, eating ham. I hadn't slept for ages.

Do you think that if they'd asked the right questions they would have kept you in hospital the first time?

I think I was doing a pretty good job of hiding it. I wanted to get out of hospital.

Do you feel you have a correct diagnosis now?

I think bipolar is closer to it. It fits in more with my symptoms. I used to feel very happy sometimes and very low at other times. I didn't need to sleep and had more energy than normal. I had times of wanting to kill myself.

But I only found out I had bipolar by looking on my record. They didn't actually *tell* me I had bipolar. My psychiatrist had it on a piece of paper and I had a sneak peek at it and I asked, 'Are they calling me bipolar now?'

Are you on medication for bipolar?

I'm on mood stabilisers and they seem to help. Now I've just got this one kind of mood. But it's hard because I don't like losing the happy side of me. I don't mind not having the down side, but I miss the ups. I used to be this laugh-all-the-time, joke-about-myself type of person. Somebody said that perhaps I had grown out of that, but how could I have grown out of something that I miss? If I'd truly grown out of it I wouldn't miss it. Now I'm just really quiet. I'm tired all the time . . . *all* the time. I don't laugh. I'm bored. I can't get involved in anything that I used to be able to . . . even computer games. I just sit here and stare into space. I have to watch what I drink and I constantly have to take medication. I'm never going to be the same girl again. I'm not a carefree young person any more. I'm a twenty-year-old who has to be responsible. I've got lots of 21st parties coming up and I'd just like to be able to have a few drinks like everyone else. I'd like to have a laugh and be goofy.

But because I have bipolar rather than schizophrenia I know I can eventually get off the medication. Schizophrenics can't ever go off their medication, but bipolar people can. I feel I already take too much medication because of my Crohn's Disease. Taking medication makes me feel different. After I take my night-time medication I'm not allowed to drive and things like that.

What do you feel has helped you most through all of this?

My friends. *All* my friends have been really supportive. They're really forgiving. They know what's happened to me and they don't judge me. They listen to me and understand what I've been through. I love my friends and I feel really appreciated when they listen to me. They also know about the bipolar and know what to do if I were to start having symptoms again. They also take me out and stuff. It gives me hope that I can come out of all of this and still have friends. It gives me hope that in the end I can just be a normal person.

I've got a psychiatrist now and a key worker and they're helping me to move on from what happened. The key worker went through a list of things that could have caused the psychosis and the stresses that were in my life (stuff like the drugs and the stuff at the funeral) so that if they come up again I know to be careful. She helps me. She's helped me to find a dietician because I said I want to lose weight. She's helping me to find housing because I said I want to move out. It's really quite good. She's like a friend and someone I can talk to about bipolar. She gives me information about it and stuff. The psychiatrist just talks about medication.

My family's also been helpful . . . supporting me, watching out for me, reassuring me.

What's happened with your boyfriend?

He's still on drugs. He's not going to change for anybody. I broke up with him but my parents would definitely warn him off if he ever came near me again. I think he'd rather find friends who'd accept the fact that he's on drugs rather than being around someone who is trying to change him. I also understand now what speed is doing to him: it's slowly aging him from the inside out. Your insides start to age. But he's going to get the wrong batch one day and die. I think he needs to go through something like I went through to bring him out of it, because he's caught.

You said early in the interview that you were screaming on the inside and nobody was listening to you. Are you still screaming on the inside?

It's muffled by the medication. I'm still depressed but it's not as bad as it was before. At the moment I don't really want to do anything except sleep . . . except when I go out with my friends. Next year I hope to go to uni or TAFE or something like that. I wanted to do something this year but then everything happened. At the moment I'm just trying to get better.

What are your thoughts when you look at everything that has happened?

In hindsight I'm a lot worse off, and I blame the drugs. I regret everything . . . I think I did the wrong thing . . . being on drugs . . . because I'm not that type of person. I never was. I was always against it. That was the way I was brought up. My friends were never on drugs.

I took dope in November and it was only completely out of my system at the end of January. The speed goes out of your system pretty quickly but the dope stays in your system for three or four months. It's stored in your fat cells somehow. I think because I was taking so much it just stayed longer.

If people take drugs, I understand why they do it, because I've taken drugs. I don't judge people. But if people knew what it could cause they might think twice. If I could warn them I would warn them. It's sad when people die.

If someone had warned you, would that have changed anything?

If someone had warned me that there was a chance of having a psychotic episode I probably wouldn't have done what I did. But I don't know . . . at the time I was convinced that what I was doing was safe.

I feel that there are a lot of people of my age experimenting with drugs. Even though I have been diagnosed with bipolar, the drugs were a big part of why I went through what I did and why it lasted so long. I hope that through my story even *some* of these people might be made aware of what could happen.

If I had any words of advice, I would say: 'Don't ever take drugs. They're not safe at all. It's not worth it. It's not worth the months in hospital. It's not worth the heartache.'

'Curiosity killed the cat.'

Curiosity got me into this . . . and then it kind of killed me a bit.

Eva

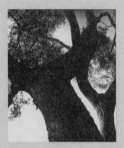

Eva is 43 years old and has suffered with phobias, anxiety and depression since her early twenties. She enjoys gardening, nature, solitude, and bushwalking. She loves the freedom of being self-employed. She likes that her obsessive perfectionism has now given way to a relaxed messiness. *'It is important for me to have a photo of a tree here. When I was suffering I often sat at the base of a wonderful old gum tree out in the bush. I called it my "mother tree". It had large roots that cradled me. Sometimes I sat under it for hours. I always came away feeling that I had taken in something of its strength, solidity and capacity for growth.'*

> Beware of desperate steps; the darkest day, lived till
> tomorrow, will have passed away.
> **William Cowper**

If I think about where I'd like to start . . . it's a moment that often comes to mind.

I was standing in the backyard with the neighbours. They'd come over for a chat. They were an older couple and they'd just been to see the movie *Shine* about the life of pianist David Helfgott. They were talking about how wonderful it was that this man with a 'mental illness' had made so much of his life.

Anyway, it was a time when I was really struggling. I spent a lot of time at home and I couldn't go out much. They so much admired this man who was 'mentally ill' and yet they were talking to someone like that right that very minute. They knew I was struggling but all they had ever been able to do was make comments that I should do more, should go on a holiday or should lose weight. Perhaps their intention was to encourage me, but I only remember feeling even worse.

Why did you feel worse?

When you have pneumonia or a broken arm people find it easy to empathise. When you're suffering from a 'mental illness' people are uncomfortable. They either tell you what to do, put a positive spin on everything or they move away. They're so busy taking care of their own discomfort that they don't see your humanity or your pain. In many ways you become completely invisible.

I also spent a lot of energy and time protecting people from their discomfort. And I probably still do. I can feel that people are sometimes uncomfortable around me. I wish I was the sort person who didn't care about that, but I'm not.

What do you do to protect them from their discomfort?

Oh . . . I hide the depth and intensity of what's going on for me. I try to act jolly even when I am screaming inside. I make an enormous effort to ask people about themselves. I steer the conversation to safe topics. As I was talking to these neighbours I was on the verge of panicking because I was trapped in the conversation, but at the same time I was still trying to make all the right noises: 'Oh really! That sounds interesting! So you feel the movie is worth seeing?' The self-control and effort required to do that, rather than to run away or fall in a heap is enormous. Sometimes a ten-minute conversation exhausted me for days afterwards. People don't understand that if they haven't been through it.

When you say that people don't see your humanity or pain, what do you mean?

Well . . . for this interview you're just sitting there listening to me. I can feel straight away that you're not putting labels, expectations, frameworks or preconceptions in front of that listening. You're just waiting to see what sort of person I am. You're interested in getting to know me. Very few people can do that when you suffer from a 'mental illness'.

Could you explain that a little more?

In dealing with people who suffer from 'mental illness', people only listen for what *they* want to hear. For instance . . . most prescribing psychiatrists will only listen to you from within the framework of psychiatry. They'll have the DSM[3] in front of them and they'll be thinking, 'Okay where can I put you and what label will I give you?' A psychiatrist would never do that if he had his wife or daughter sitting in front of him and in distress. The psychiatrist doesn't listen to the patient's distress he's only trying to find somewhere to fit you in *his* map of the world.

They probably need labels so they can fill in a gap on a piece of paper, but those labels shouldn't get in the way of the human beings involved. I just don't think that psychiatric diagnoses are the same as diagnoses like 'broken pelvis' and 'arthritis'. I've been given different diagnoses at different times in my life, simply because I was dealing with different issues and was distressed in different ways . . . just like anyone else would be. For instance, if someone close to you dies, your distress would be different to the distress if you lost an earring.

I once saw a very funny paper that someone had

---

3   Diagnostic and Statistical Manual of Mental Disorders. The DSM is the main classification of 'mental disorders' used by psychiatrists.

written about a new disorder. It was called something like 'Compulsive Labelling Disorder'. It was written just like the DSM and it was mocking psychiatrists who label. But it made its point too – labels are just *so* arbitrary. You can call anything a 'disorder' and find a set of criteria to justify the label.

Labels also make it really hard to keep your sense of self intact. You have to keep reminding yourself that you're a human being and more than just a label.

What is a 'human being' then?

It's everything. All of what makes up who people are. Feelings, thoughts, body, spirit, soul, hopes, dreams, character, qualities . . . everything. The mental health system only tends to treat your body. It treats the whole 'mental illness' thing as some sort of technical exercise in brain chemistry. That is utterly dehumanising.

I remember once going for an initial assessment with a psychiatrist. He asked all sorts of questions about my past, about my feelings, about my relationships . . . and while he was asking them, I felt a sense of relief. I thought, 'Wow, this guy is actually going to take *all* these things into account!' But then when he finished he simply said, 'You have a chemical imbalance in your brain and perhaps also some genetic involvement.' And I thought, '*What?!*' I felt so diminished. I'd shared my feelings, my doubts, my hopes, my life . . . and with a dash of his pen I had a prescription for pills. Utter invalidation! He'd reduced my whole life to chemical imbalance and pills. And what's even weirder is that of all the times I've been told I have some chemical imbalance or some genetic predisposition, nobody has *ever* done a test. It's pure theory. It's supposition. They wouldn't diagnose liver disease or a stomach ulcer or a broken arm without doing tests and X-rays.

I think the mental health system has to be a moral exercise rather than a technical one.

What do you mean by moral exercise?

I'm not exactly sure moral is the right word, but stuff like ... What is people's experience of suffering and how can it be alleviated in a way that allows them to flourish? What does it mean to lead a good life? A meaningful life? How can people be treated with compassion and have their personal meanings validated? It's even just asking stuff like, 'What's a human being?' There's so much stuff there ... When you have prescribing psychiatrists at the helm of the mental health system those sorts of questions will be mostly ignored. I am sure there are good kindly people out there who are also psychiatrists, but the mental health system must do more than just fix people up a bit, get them through a crisis and then hope that they shut up. We're a lot more complex than that.

Lately there has been a movement to employ peer support workers in the mental health system. They're recruiting people who have been diagnosed with a 'mental illness' but are 'stable' to help people who are currently going through crises. That all sounds really good in principle, but the problem is that they're only choosing and then educating people along the lines of the prescribing psychiatrists. There's only one point of view: 'Stay on your medication and all will be well.' It's all medical model. That's really limiting. There's so much more to life and people and relationships.

How do you think the mental health system could be changed?

Well ... people talk a lot about funding – more funding for more services. But what sorts of services? The services that the mental health system offers have not helped me in any way in the *long* term and I think that applies to *many* people. You have to look *outside* the mental health system to get the services that you really need. The main service should be some sort of *long*-term psychotherapy. That's what has helped me. You can get that sort of service from counsellors, from talking psychiatrists, psychotherapists . . . but you have to go *outside* the system.

It's really interesting . . . in the news coverage of that mining rescue in Beaconsfield, Tasmania, there was talk that the miners would need counselling and ongoing support. Even the kids in the local schools were given counselling. But then its pretty weird when you consider that the mental health system doesn't provide *any* ongoing counselling and psychotherapy for people who may have been traumatised for years and years and years . . . not just for two weeks. Just imagine the outcry if someone said that any problems those miners might have is simply due to brain chemistry!

What do you feel is helpful about psychotherapy?

Well . . . firstly I think you *need* to ask what 'mental illness' actually is. Nobody asks that question! I think most 'mental illness' is what happens to a human being who has been traumatised and has not had the resources either inside or outside to understand what has happened. I think if you look at a person with 'mental illness' and realise, 'this person has been utterly traumatised at some point in their lives and they need help to cope with it', then something changes. People aren't 'mentally ill' . . . they don't have something wrong with the chemicals in their brains . . . they're traumatised! Their whole body, mind, spirit, soul, behaviour is simply *reflecting* that trauma. You can try to fix behaviour, or body or whatever else, but it does nothing to address the deeper issues.

I remember once going to a hospital emergency ward after a bad fall on a bushwalk and they happened to put me in the bed next to the psychiatric bed. It was really interesting to lie there as an observer and watch the way the psychiatric patients were treated by some of the nursing staff. It was horrendous. They were treated like naughty children. They were treated like they were a nuisance and a pest, and were just there to waste the time of the staff. It was *so* obvious to me that these people were traumatised and were trying desperately to make sense of overwhelming 'stuff' inside. But then they were treated so abysmally that they were really just being double-traumatised.

So you believe the treatment they received was just adding to their distress.

Yeah. Absolutely. There's a way in which professional people put people with a 'mental illness' into catch-22 positions, and create environments that are in many ways similar to those that traumatised them. They're no-win situations.

Could you give an example?

I remember a psychiatrist once toying with whether to put the word 'psychotic' on my file. It was like a technical exercise for him. He didn't agree with something I'd said and so he was almost using the label of 'psychotic' as leverage. I could suss out straightaway that it was some sort of power struggle. The implication was, 'You have to be careful what you say to me because I can do whatever I want.' I thought what I'd said to him was absolutely valid . . . but I knew that if I complained or got angry with his use of the word 'psychotic', he would have all the justification he needed to put it on my file. I had to play *his* game . . . and that game *really* was crazy! You have to be *so* careful all the time that you remain even, nice, pleasant . . . if you get angry or upset they don't see that you're just as entitled to your anger as the rest of the population. They'll give it all sorts of names . . . from psychosis to paranoia to 'denial' . . . you'll become 'disruptive', 'non-compliant'.

So you believe that psychotherapy could offer something different to this?

Yes. Definitely. Psychotherapy can offer traumatised people *so* much. Firstly, it enables you to begin to put your life into some sort of context. You can begin to understand what happened in the past. You can work through and feel the traumatic events of your life so that they no longer overwhelm every living moment. You can begin to understand your life in terms of the past, present and future. You can begin to work out what stuff belongs in the past, what stuff you have to deal with now and then you can begin to work out where you're going and what you want from life. You can begin to realise that you are a valuable human being. And most importantly you can get in touch with who you most truly are and realise that it is okay to be who you are. That's the crux of mental illness I think: *you don't feel you have any right to be who you are.*

In what way does therapy allow you to realise that you have a right to be yourself?

I think it's in the relationship. A therapist has to be someone who's not scared of developing a deep, caring and long-term relationship with you. You have to feel a sense of connection . . . and it has to be a two-way thing. A therapist can't just *pretend* to listen or *pretend* to care just because they're taught to do that in the text books. The client will suss that out straight away. When you're deeply cared for, when all of who you are is deeply accepted and is okay with someone else, when you can say whatever you want and it will be taken seriously and regarded as *meaningful*, you start to feel okay with yourself. You get in touch with who you really are.

It's not about techniques . . . whether pills or psychological games like CBT[4] or whatever. These things can certainly be small steps along the way, but the suffering that is called 'mental illness' is a lot deeper and more intense than that and so it has to be addressed at that deeper level. If people don't feel that they have a right to be themselves, any changes in behaviour or thinking or biochemistry aren't going to fix anything in the long term.

What do you mean when you speak of getting in touch with who you truly are?

I suppose it's spiritual stuff. It's like I feel something inside that is really *who I am*. It's something I feel in my gut. When I'm in touch with that, it's like I can speak and act and it's really *me* coming out into the world. It's like listening to my own internal rhythms and then following them. It's like knowing what's right for me. It's like I'm the authority in my own existence. It feels right. It feels solid. I feel connected to deeper parts of myself that others might call soul, spirit or God. When I'm in touch with that, life feels good. I feel at home in myself. It's the opposite of 'mental illness'. I can still get knocked around but I don't crash.

You said earlier that you feel people are traumatised rather than 'mentally ill' . . .

Yes. I didn't have an 'illness'. As soon as you call it an 'illness' it sweeps away the reality of what happened. There's also an implication in those words that I have a disease or that there's something wrong with me. There's

---

4   Cognitive Behaviour Therapy

nothing wrong with me. I believe that to be true for the vast majority of people.

. . . and it's not even maladjustment. I remember going to GROW groups and they spoke of maladjustment. But it's not . . . it's a *perfect* adjustment. I had adjusted *perfectly* to the environment of my childhood.

. . . when you speak of trauma, are you speaking of child abuse?

In my case, yes. But trauma can be anything . . . a break-up of a relationship, loss, death of a loved one, torture, war experiences, mining accidents . . . anything can be traumatic for the person involved. And it's not up to psychiatrists or psychologists or doctors to judge what's traumatic and what's not . . . it's completely subjective. If a person *feels* traumatised then they are. And trauma can't be judged like some numerical equation. What's traumatic for one person isn't necessarily traumatic for another. There's been so much coverage of sexual abuse in the media, as though by its 'sexual' nature it is the only sort of abuse or trauma that is bad enough to be damaging. But *any* sort of abuse can be damaging . . . even something that others might not even blink an eye at.

I think for me it was a bit like someone coming from Rwanda and getting plonked into an Australian environment. People would think it was quite normal if a person from Rwanda didn't know how to speak English straight away or cook the perfect Aussie barbecue. People wouldn't immediately expect him or her to know all the rules and behave like a perfect Australian.

But I was coming from my own 'Rwanda'. I was coming from an alien environment into the everyday world. It would be horrifying to think that someone from Rwanda might be labelled as 'mentally ill' just because they couldn't do everything in 'correct' or socially acceptable ways and started to get confused and upset. It would be even worse if this person had also been traumatised in a civil war and was still terrified of loud noises and was then medicated or given further labels. And what if he or she complained about their treatment but such complaints were only seen as part of the 'mental illness' and he or she was then branded as 'difficult', 'defiant' or 'disruptive'? And what if this person was actually asking for help and asking to be listened to and guided, but that guidance simply wasn't available or only came in the form of medication?

If people are given validation, are listened to, are understood and supported then they can get through anything.

Everything I became – the panic attacks, the phobias, the crippling anxiety, the depression, the fear, the suicidality – makes sense when I see it in the light of what happened to me as a child. It is *utterly* meaningful. And it wasn't just incidents of abuse, even though those were certainly there. It was the whole kit and caboodle . . . it was the whole tone of my upbringing. I really felt, and at times still feel, that I don't have any right to be me.

What happened in your childhood that left you with the feeling that you could not be yourself?

Well firstly, if you're abused in some way, then you are treated like an object . . . a nothing . . . an outer shell with nothing inside. If you're treated like an object as a child then that's what you believe you are. You can't abuse someone unless you totally deny that person his or her humanity.

My father and mother both lived with the legacy of growing up in the Second World War. Many family members were killed. They both reacted to that in their own ways. My mother was quite cold and distant and my father was very authoritarian and abusive. I always had to do whatever my father said and I had very little sense of acting, speaking and being in the world beyond that. If you live in that sort of environment when you're a kid you can't suddenly develop autonomy when you're an adult . . . and if as a kid you have a roof over your head and go to school, you're made to feel guilty that you're even alive . . . you're told to be grateful for everything . . . if you cry you're told that they had it much worse . . . I sometimes wonder what's going to happen to the second and third generations of the war in Iraq . . . because it gets passed on . . .

I lived with a certain level of anxiety *the whole time.* I never knew when my father would explode. I also never knew when my mother would turn against me. There was always a sense that she was my ally when he wasn't home, but that she would turn against me when he *was* home. Rules changed all the time to suit my parents and their moods. There were mixed messages, there were no-win situations, hypocrisy, incongruence, vicious name-calling, violence. That sort of stuff is utterly devastating and crazy-making for a kid. There's nothing solid to bounce off so you don't develop any solidity within.

Also, I never remember my parents having a conversation with me. That affects me to this day. Other people have an ease with words; they can chat back and forth without being overwhelmed. It's hard to explain because people say I'm articulate, but the struggle that goes on behind the scenes is enormous. I really struggle with finding the right words and I still find it difficult to believe that anything I say is valid.

Love was conditional. I always had to perform to get the love I craved and so I've always felt an enormous anxiety about whether I am performing okay. I feel reasonably confident in social situations now, but there's still an element of 'Did I do it okay? Did I seem *normal?*' If I'm concerned whether I'm fitting in and doing okay in social situations I'll still check it out with my husband. The one way I could please my parents and get a sense of being loved was to be neat and tidy and get good marks in school. They would boast to their friends how clever I was but on another day hit me and tell me I was being 'too clever'. I became an extreme and obsessive perfectionist . . . about everything . . . a control freak I guess.

And there was just plain fear. I lived with fear from the word go. The world always felt really unsafe. I didn't feel safe. Ever. I remember happy times in my childhood but if I get an overall feeling it's just a sense of being scared and of the world being a really dangerous place. I didn't realise there was any other way to live until I was an adult . . . and by then everything I had learnt no longer applied. All I knew was a set of rules that would keep me as safe as possible but they weren't rules that fitted into the everyday world.

I found the everyday world unmanageable and over-whelming and I didn't understand what was going on. It didn't make sense to me. Kids at school used to call me 'Starer' or 'The Block' because I couldn't interact. All the other kids seemed to know rules and ways of playing and being with each other that I didn't. I remember just being this little girl who was so rigid and tight and awkward and confused. The only rules I knew were 'not to say too much', 'not do anything to bring attention to myself' and 'to do what other people told me to do'. I was trying so hard just to be good and to be what everyone else wanted me to be that I never learnt to be *myself.* I never felt acceptable inside. I always felt like it was best to be a sort of non-person.

In my early twenties when I was trying to find my place in the world I just didn't have any 'me' inside to be able to cope with it all. I broke down.

Could you tell me more about breaking down?

I suppose it was more like a downhill spiral. I just got deeper and deeper into a pit of utter utter fear. The fear was so awful. *Every* day. *All* day. It started with panic attacks and then I started to fear the panic attacks. Then I started to fear the situations in which I panicked. Bit by bit I stopped being able to do anything. I'd run out of shops. I'd run home if I was out on a walk. Eventually I couldn't go to the shops, banks, picture theatres, walk across a car park, drive, talk to people . . . there were a couple of years when I couldn't even go to the letter box. There was even a time when walking down the hallway was scary. I was agoraphobic, claustrophobic, everything phobic . . . I was so scared of being trapped in *any situation*. I spent most of my time negotiating with myself how I could escape from every conceivable situation. It took over every moment of my life.

And then I started to worry . . . I worried incessantly about anything, but particularly something in the future. Making an appointment made me very ill. I'd only make an appointment on the spur of the moment or if I had a dreadful toothache or was really sick. But I'd worry about *anything* whatsoever: tree branches falling on my head, doctors prescribing the wrong medication, the brakes in my car giving out, having cancer or some life-threatening illness, the roof coming off in a storm, my husband leaving, getting electrocuted, getting bitten by a spider, people killing me in my sleep. It was *everything*.

There were also times when I couldn't eat. Other people had to eat from the sugar before me in case someone had put some poisonous powder in there. I couldn't eat food at restaurants because someone might have poisoned my food or not taken care to see whether something was past its use-by date. I always had to cook food myself and check out all the items very carefully. I checked all containers and bags from the supermarket to see if they were airtight or still fully sealed. If they weren't, I threw them out. There were all these safety measures that I had to put in place before I could eat.

I remember a friend inviting me over to dinner one night and she had cooked a dish with mushrooms. During the course of the dinner I became convinced that the mushrooms were actually poisonous . . . but I still continued to eat them because I didn't want to hurt her feelings. With every bite I took, I thought it would be my last . . . and then I still tried to make polite conversation. The hell of making someone else's feelings more important than my own *life* was horrendous. I was exhausted for weeks afterwards; completely and utterly wrecked. It felt like I'd had someone holding a gun to my head. I know I was 'doing it to myself' but the trauma wasn't any less.

I came to fear everything . . . everything became dangerous. *Everything.* At night I checked under the bed. In the bed. I needed to control absolutely everything. I came to fear people. I was paranoid that everyone was watching me. I couldn't function at all.

Eventually the only way I could deal with life was to think the absolute worst in every situation and then deal with it that way. I didn't dare to hope.

I also had bouts of depression and suicidality that lasted many months. They were times that I just didn't want to be alive and I thought of death endlessly. A few times I drove my car down really steep roads, and I thought, 'Well if there's a God and I'm meant to be

alive, then I'll be okay, but if there isn't, well I'll die.'
I slashed my wrists a couple of times and also self-
mutilated a *lot* when the pain was really bad. People
see self-mutilation as a pretty crazy thing to do, but it
actually makes a lot of sense, and often kept me safe.
I'd hit myself with rocks, scrape myself until I bled . . .
other things as well.

How did self-mutilation make sense?

When there was dreadful emotional pain, physical
pain was a relief. It actually stopped me from going
into suicidal stuff. I had been quite used to physical pain
in my childhood, and I understood it more than emotional pain. I had also been abused for crying or getting
angry and so my only way of dealing adequately with
my feelings was to do what my parents did: abuse.

In their own way, sometimes the blood and bruises
were even joyous.

Why was that?

. . . when I had a weeping open wound I had a way
of taking care of myself . . . emotional and spiritual
wounds are so complicated . . . physical wounds are
easy . . . you wash them carefully, put some antiseptic
on them, put a little bandage on . . . it was the only
time my mother was really gentle and careful with me
and even now I just love the smell of bandaids and
bandages and Elastoplast. I feel at home and cared for
and loved. When I had a bandage somewhere, I could
love and care for myself. I remember once I had self-
inflicted gashes down my leg and the neighbours came
over and saw them. They were horrified and asked what
I had done. I said I had been digging in the garden and
had gashed my leg with the hoe. In that instant they
stopped telling me what to do, they seemed to care, they
were interested in *me* . . . and I didn't panic. I felt human.

I'd also like to mention that there were times when I was really quite violent. In reality I am the most non-violent person you can imagine, but I *was* at times violent. I'm not proud of those episodes but I think they're worth mentioning. I would just totally lose it. The violence would mostly be aimed at myself or something inanimate but also occasionally at my husband. I wrecked a lot of things. Threw things around. Gradually I did develop self-control. I bought these big old ugly furry toys at a local second-hand shop and I'd 'kill' them. I learnt to understand the violence and learnt better ways of dealing it.

Why is it important for you to mention about the violence?

Violence and 'mental illness' are often tied together in the media; people lump them together. Professionals also tend to dismiss it as, 'Oh, she's simply acting out'. I think I'd internalised a lot of my father's violence, but the violence and 'acting out' also came about when I felt I wasn't being listened to. If you're trying to find your voice, if you're trying to find out who you are, and then people don't listen to you it is insane inside. It is hell on earth. It feels like you're just getting a tiny sense of something that might be solid, and then it gets trodden on.

I also think that if you go quietly up to someone and say, 'Hey things are really bad today,' they don't take you seriously. Sometimes you just *have* to scream before someone takes any notice. So often I used to wish that people took notice *before* I screamed.

I know it must be hard for people, but listening is vital. If people can't listen they should say, 'Look I haven't got the time right now, but can we talk in an hour?' Clear boundaries would have been fine with me . . .

they're much better than being discarded or dismissed. I feel that so much violence in people with 'mental illness' is as a result of not being listened to. It is *such* a frustration. People treat you like a moron. An idiot. *All* people need to be listened to, but when you're suffering, that need is doubled . . . tripled. I can't stress the importance of listening enough. *Real* listening . . . and it shouldn't just be to the noisy and loud voices. It should be to the quiet voices too.

I think Lifeline[5] is really good in that respect. If you ring Lifeline, they *listen.* If you're feeling suicidal or if you're feeling crazy, they *listen!* They don't put their own points of view in your face. They don't manage or assess you like some soulless piece of meat. Having someone anonymous on the other side of the phone, who will simply allow you to talk and allow you to put things into some sort of perspective, has been *so* important to me. There are some Lifeline counsellors who aren't all that great, but a lot of them are excellent.

You've mentioned medication a number of times through the interview. What is your opinion of the medications you were given?

Hopeless.

Could you go into a little more detail?

I thought medication was horrendous. They only used it because they didn't know what else to do with me. And I hated the side effects. Medication always put a wall between me and the rest of the world. It was like I was operating at so much less than I am. Certainly some of the anxiety and pain was dulled but I found it awful. I never want to live my life around them again.

---

5   A 24-hour crisis telephone counselling service operating throughout Australia. Phone 131114.

With the first antidepressants I was on I had a dry mouth, constipation, nightmares, blurred vision and a sense of unreality ... all of which only made my anxiety and panic attacks worse and made me feel like everything was even more hopeless. There were others and a number of times I simply refused to take pills ... anti-psychotics, mood stabilisers ... because of the massive side effects and the fact that it seemed to just be a way of filling in time in an appointment ... Sometimes I just felt that they wanted to be seen to be doing *something*. I had a dreadful gastric reaction to the last one I took and I lost something like ten kilos in three weeks. I had to stop taking it. My gut took a long time to recuperate. And then the psychiatrist still said that I must have had a gastro bug! They don't believe you because you're a psychiatric patient. They don't take you seriously when you complain. Just because you're suffering and traumatised they assume you don't know your own body. That is such bullshit. It makes me really angry. I am intelligent, I have insight ... treat me with respect! I do occasionally take sleeping pills and some Valium when I'm anxious. That's enough. I never take any more than I need to because I don't want to get hooked. I get them from my GP.

Where are you in your life now?

For the first time I feel okay for this point in my life. I feel reasonably solid and at times I feel quite content. I still think I've probably got a way to go but I think I'm doing okay for now. For the first time in a very long time I don't have a regular counsellor, psychiatrist or therapist in my life.

Has that sense of solidity come about solely through psychotherapy?

That was a big part of it for a *long* time. I am so grateful for the therapists who took me from those very dark times . . . who stood by me and walked the nightmare with me . . . but there is so much else . . . it *all* adds up. You *learn* from *all* the bits and pieces along the way . . . I see my life like a journey and that journey never ends. I think when you've been through really hard times and you get through them you begin to realise that. When you're on a journey or on a trip, things *can* get really difficult. You might only be travelling to Paris or something, but things *can* go wrong: you're delayed in Singapore, you have to wait in long queues, your taxi driver is a maniac, you lose your luggage . . . but in the end you get to Paris . . . and it's worth it. All the difficult stuff that happened is *part* of it. You don't expect it to go perfectly. When that happens in your day-to-day life, you become more resilient . . . you stretch the boundaries of who you know yourself to be . . . you go with the flow more . . . but you can only really start to do that when you feel some solidity inside.

What were the other 'bits and pieces'?

Along with therapy I explored *everything*: I read a lot, explored spiritual stuff, learnt a lot from animals, *loved* nature and began to use my body. I learnt that some days it was enough to take in the sun shining on the leaves or the beauty of a flower . . . I began to think that the world also needs the gentle and sensitive people to notice the beautiful things. I didn't want to be one of the busy people.

I also began to really feel the reality of the world of spirit and soul. I felt that I was a part of something much bigger and didn't feel so isolated any more.

How did that become a reality in your life?

I'm not exactly sure. I didn't just 'get it' one day. I'd always looked to spiritual things. I'd read books . . .

been to classes ... talked to people. I've never liked conventional religion ... sin and judgement don't appeal to me ... it's too much like my parents. I also don't put much faith in people who are popes or gurus. And that fundamentalist emotional waving of the hands doesn't appeal to me either ... you can whip anyone up into an emotional frenzy but it's not real and solid and deep inside.

Things just slowly started to add up ... I realised that when I really took in a sunset for instance, it was a spiritual experience. It was as though I took in something of the quality of the sunset and came away a bigger person. And then I realised I could do that with lots of things ... even people ... I wasn't closing off from them ... and as a result I wasn't closing off so much from myself ... I wasn't dismissing people or situations ... I was taking them in and becoming bigger ... and just lately I've begun to feel compassion. That's *big*, that's *massive*. It's almost like an answer, but not an answer you could just present someone with: 'Be compassionate and all your worries will be over.' That's the sort of thing psychology and the New Age stuff do. I don't think you can really change anything on a deep level by a simple decision to do so. Those things work for two weeks and then fall in a heap.

Only recently I have begun to feel the vastness of who I am inside – my soul – and also the vastness of the physical world. In every moment I know I can step into that world in a way of my choosing and in a way that I am expressing that soul as best I can. But it's also about not giving myself a hard time if I'm shitty, upset or once again struggling! It's all part of it.

I guess the big thing is that I don't struggle against the struggle any more ... and as a result I don't *suffer*.

And it's also about saying 'no' to things.

What might you say 'no' to?

It can be something quite trivial like a computer game. When I was suffering I spent a lot of time playing endless computer games. It passed the time and the repetition eased my anxiety. Sometimes I start to play a game now, and I know it's just a habit. It's something that can drag me down . . . so I would rather choose to sit and do nothing until I can listen for what is right. But some of the 'no's' have also been pretty big ones . . . saying 'no' to people when I'm busy or need time for myself . . . also saying, 'No, you cannot treat me that way.'

And it's saying 'no' to a particular view of life that's so very one-sided. It's the sort of stuff the media goes on with . . . wrinkle-free, slim, good-looking, happy lives . . . that leads to so much suffering and anxiety in people. Psychiatry also perpetuates that. It draws a circle around all the pretty, happy and nice stuff, calls it 'normal' or 'socially acceptable' and then tries to medicate away anything that's outside the circle. There's no room for eccentricity and difference.

Life comes in all colours, all shades, all sizes, and all textures. Frankly some of the sanest people I have ever met were those who have been labelled as 'mentally ill'. And some of the truly scariest people I have ever met have passed themselves off as quite admirably normal.

How do you account for that?

I think that when you're suffering and you don't fit in, you ask questions and you try to find answers . . . *real* answers. The result is that you end up with *real* people. That's all I've ever really wanted . . . a real life.

And you have that?

I'm getting there.

George

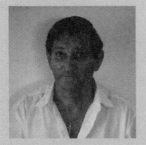

George is 62 years old and has suffered from obsessive compulsive disorder (OCD) since the age of fourteen. He spent his early life in England, Egypt and Malta and immigrated to Australia in his twenties. He is married and has two adult children. He enjoys music, playing trumpet and cornet in a band and working on the computer. *'I would like my photo included here. I believe that it is important to leave something behind – a legacy. If there is one thing that is important for me to bring out through this interview, it is to save the children. Take care of the children for they are our future. Please take care of the children.'*

Early memories

My mother was Maltese, but from Egypt, and my father was a regimental sergeant major in the British Army. They met in Cairo. My father was at both Normandy and Dunkirk. I was born in Sussex, England, during a very bad time in the Second World War. There were frequent bombings and the Doodlebugs – the German unmanned rockets – frequently whined overhead. As a result I was kept inside a lot.

I would describe my mother as a very loving and devoted woman. Although she was a strong-willed woman, she had a very hard time in the war. I believe that as a result of this she was often quite anxious. She also had very bad eyesight. Because of her sight, she didn't notice that I had contracted rickets through lack of sunshine. A nurse told her that if she didn't take me outside soon, I would die. I was given artificial sunlight treatment and I had splints put on my legs. However, as a result of my illness, my father was posted out to Malta. My mother's origins were Maltese, so that pleased her immensely. We went to Malta and my rickets disappeared.

I was actually lost for three hours in Malta. Mum said afterwards that she gave me a good smack, which I now feel wouldn't have been the appropriate thing to do. I'm not sure what actually happened during this time, but what comes back to me now is that even at this young age, I had enormous feelings of guilt.

Then in 1948 we went to Egypt. This made my mother very happy because her family lived in Egypt. Although life was basically good I was very anxious. I wonder if it was the fact that I had very bad eyesight like my mother and it hadn't been picked up. It wasn't until one day I was run over by an Egyptian man on a bicycle, that a teacher suggested I might need glasses. I remember being cut from head to foot and the nuns attending to my dressings. But I continued to feel very nervous and I could never quite put my finger on it. I used to bite my fingernails right down till they bled.

I suppose there are incidents or traumas that affected me as I grew up. For instance, I always had a feeling that if anyone touched me around the neck I would go crazy. Only later did I find out that my brother nearly strangled me with a bit of rope when I was a child. Perhaps that event was unresolved. Afterwards I had very severe nightmares and would wake up screaming and sweating profusely. Eventually that eased off, but I was still very nervous.

Because of surgery my mother had incontinence much of her life, and so she used to come into the toilet or bathroom when we were in there. I assumed that it was just normal for males and females to be in together. One day my father punished me and dressed me up in a girl's dress and paraded me in front of the family because he considered, incorrectly, that I had been playing around near the girls' toilets.

However, the time in Egypt was fairly secure for me. Eventually though, the English were asked to leave the country by King Fuhad. The British prime minister at the time, Anthony Eden, agreed to this. The children and the mothers were the first to go. Dad went with Mum because of her sight. In 1952 we returned to England in quite a hurried exit. As we came into the docks at Southampton we were told that King George VI had died that very evening.

Once we were back in England we went to live in Y . . . I was happy there, but continued to be very nervous. I was called 'highly strung' and got excited very easily. I couldn't sit still. They called me 'The Willick'. I wonder if I had a mild form of OCD at this stage, but what I would call a healthy form. Rather than worry about germs, repeat myself, check doors, count numbers or whatever, I would continually whistle and sing the same thing over and over.

I loved my mother and I *did* love my father at this stage.

By 1953 Dad had left the army and we got a council house.

The beginning

An event happened in Y . . . that changed my life. I got involved with a boy and his sister in a sexually very innocent childish way. When the mother of the girl asked me about it, I honestly owned up. She came and reported it to my parents. Mum smacked me across the face. My father said, 'Don't you worry, after this is all over, I'm going to get you,' meaning that he was going to give me the belt. I took my punishment and it hurt me, but then I started to worry about whether I would do it again . . . and I couldn't stop worrying about it. I kept thinking that I might do it again.

Although my father had always been a very intimidating presence in my life, my relationship with him up to this point had been on a fairly good basis. I had been hit before, but not heavy-handedly. In relation to this incident however, he had been very threatening, and I wasn't used to being threatened in this way by someone I really loved. That was very traumatic to me. His threat deeply hurt me and disturbed me. If he had counselled me or talked with me about the incident it would have been different.

We moved to our own house. I had begun to suffer from depression occasionally, though not really bad depression. And I suffered a lot from insecurity and anxiety. I remember one night when my parents went out, my brother said to me jokingly, 'I'm going to kill you tonight.' I was a very sensitive person and I took him seriously. I was very frightened. He eventually realised the impact it had on me and said he was sorry.

I went to secondary modern school and it was a good time in my life. I was sleeping well and had a good appetite. I was still nervous and a bit depressed but it was a good time. Then I left school at the age of fourteen and a half, and that was when my life turned.

Like everyone else I had always had the fear of losing my parents. It used to worry me. Then two weeks after starting work I went to the pictures and on the way there I saw a church. I had always feared death. I had been able to smell it. And I could never understand why. Anyway, this particular day, I imagined my mother lying dead in this church and then all of a sudden came the thought of doing something bad . . . *killing my mother.* There was no motivation, it was simply the thought of actually doing it. That was traumatic. Very traumatic. It was as though somebody was standing with a gun at my head. I would start to rid myself of the thought but it only came back again. It went over and over and over. (I now relate this incident to the innocent sexual business with the girl – of fearing that I would do it again.)

I got home and even though my mother had bad sight she sensed that there was something different about me. She asked me what was wrong. I said, 'I can't tell you.' I was crying. Eventually I told her and she said, 'Oh that's just silly.' She said, 'Here's a knife. I know you wouldn't do that.' I said, 'I know, but I just can't get rid of the thought.'

She suggested I talk to the family doctor and tell the priest in confession. I went and told the priest. He gave me penance. I went to the doctor. He said I had a 'brain disturbance' – or in other words a breakdown . . . and he put me on some tablets. I must make the point that in those days taking tablets was a sign of weakness, especially when it came to mental illness. If you couldn't control your thoughts or your behaviour, you were a bad person. Anyway, the doctor referred me to the psychiatrist at Y . . . hospital, but the thoughts only got worse and worse and eventually he talked of sending me to a place everyone called the madhouse.

The thing about this illness, as with any illness, is that it has to be treated straightaway. If it is treated straightaway, I think the impact on the life of the sufferer would be a hell of a lot less. My biggest problem was that when I was young there was such a stigma. There was the stigma of having something wrong with your mind and not being in control. A mental illness in those days was also a big shame on the family; it reflected on the whole family image. Added to that was the fact that there was no real family interaction or support because of the lack of understanding of these disorders. I stopped seeing the psychiatrist because I didn't want this stigma and I was frightened of being sent away.

But I continued to obsess about killing my mother. And then it simply transferred onto other things. It became a fear of doing anything wrong: of stealing, assaulting another child. It went onto everything. It wasn't the fact that I *wanted* to do any of these things, it was the *fear* of doing them that was the problem. To cut a long story short I started going into a decline. I started a mild form of self-mutilation – deliberately tensing my neck and making my breathing very shallow. I was continually tense in my throat and also had rounded shoulders. I did a welding course and I shook the whole time. Even my feet were shaking.

My self-esteem was very low. When you have good self-esteem, when your self-esteem is intact, no matter if you have lost a leg or lost an arm or become a quadriplegic, you can live with it. I remember that movie, *The Elephant Man*. He was happy with himself even though he was the Elephant Man! When something affects your self-esteem you start to doubt things, you start to get paranoid about people looking at you, pointing their finger at you. You start to imagine all kinds of things that are very disturbing and very painful. You lose confidence in yourself. You don't want to go out any more. And then when you start going down the road of self-mutilation your life becomes a complete mess. It is *so* painful mentally and emotionally. I can't explain it.

Only later did I understand my fear of death and the smell of death. Down the hill from where we had lived in Malta was the hospital and at the back of that hospital was the mortuary. My mother used to take us in there as small children, whenever she paid respects to someone who had died. I hadn't remembered that.

In all of this, the best therapy was playing soccer. It released everything.

Finding the words

By the time I reached my twenties I was very depressed. I was very frightened to go out with women. I heard my parents' voices: 'don't touch', 'you fool'. My self-esteem was very low. I was nothing. Nobody. I thought my problems would disappear if I came to Australia. My sister had already moved here and my parents had followed.

But of course nothing changed. My environment had changed but not my brain.

When I got married the same thing just carried on and on. And then I started having 'the doubt'. Had I shut the door? Had I turned the kettle off? Checking. Checking. Counting numbers. Counting numbers. I wanted to see every numberplate when I was driving. Ruminating over and over. Then I had children and I couldn't touch them. I couldn't bathe them. I had the fear of hurting them. I had the fear of cot death.

Psychiatry didn't help me. They didn't explain anything to me. A psychiatrist would speak to me and then they would take out their prescription pad and put me on tranquillisers. But I couldn't take the tranquillisers. How can you be sedated when you're trying to work a job in which you have to cut steel to a tolerance of half a millimetre? They also gave me an SSRI[6] and then an MAOI[7]. Those made me feel either nauseous or brought my blood pressure so far down that I was on the point of passing out.

I had a whole day of tests at a psychiatric hospital and they come to the conclusion that I had slight paranoia. I already knew I had a touch of paranoia because I used to think people were looking at me. I did some hypnotherapy and relaxation. I went to a private hospital to have insulin treatment for three weeks and that was a waste of time. All in all low doses of Valium were best because they quietened my mind and allowed me to concentrate . . . but it wasn't enough.

By this time I was making mistakes at work. I couldn't concentrate because my thoughts were continually going over and over like a broken record.

After seeing many doctors my biggest breakthrough came when I saw a psychiatrist as an outpatient. I explained everything to him and he said, 'I know what you've got, you've got Obsessions'. They didn't call it OCD then. He told me I would probably need medication for the rest of my life, but all the same it was good to have the diagnosis. It told me why I was like I was. I had been trying to tell people about it all my life, but nobody would really listen. I had never been able to communicate what was wrong with me. Now, at least, I had the words.

---

6   Selective serotonin reuptake inhibitor. A class of antidepressant drugs that may be used to treat depression and anxiety disorders. SSRIs help to increase the levels of the neurotransmitter serotonin.

7   Monoamine oxidase inhibitor. A particularly powerful class of antidepressant drugs often used sparingly because of quite lethal drug and food interactions. MAOIs may be used for depression, agoraphobia and social anxiety. They prevent the breakdown of the neurotransmitter monoamine.

Swallowing

One day I went into a health food shop. There was a bottle on the shelf called Nerve Tonic. Within two tablespoons I had instant relief. I had confidence. A quiet mind. I didn't feel any fear. It was wonderful. I was on that for twenty years. I still didn't lead a normal life, but all the same I could go to the show, I could concentrate more, I was making less mistakes at work, I felt more confident and I could sleep. Before that I would lie awake worrying, worrying, worrying.

And then because I was feeling better, I decided to become a volunteer for St John Ambulance. I started going out as third man with the ambulance team. What I didn't realise though, is that because I had been taking the Nerve Tonic for so long, the therapeutic properties had begun to wear off. I was getting really nervous and I knew I was. But I kept forcing myself to go against my instincts and the way I felt. I was trying to make myself look good in the eyes of my parents, even though they weren't even vaguely interested in what I was doing. The worst place was the morgue of course . . . and undressing the deceased. I never saw anything really bad like dead children, thank God, but it upset me all the same.

And then slowly something started to happen to me . . . and I didn't realise it. I would start to eat a meal and then I couldn't swallow. And it got worse and worse. I became frightened stiff of swallowing and then I *knew* it was time to get out of St John. And I've been frightened ever since. Swallowing is my biggest problem. But it was my own fault. I'd already had anxiety from an early age and by doing St John I had thrown myself into the deep end. It was *so* stupid. And I continued to do it to please my parents. People choose career paths because they are trying to please someone else and then they end up having breakdowns. If people follow their own path they'll enjoy life a lot more.

I wonder whether the fear of swallowing was in the back of my mind because of the rope – because it wasn't treated. I wonder whether it resurfaced. I even had a fear of breathing at that time. It sounds silly and irrational, because a baby eats and breathes naturally. But the reason they don't have such a fear, is that they have their mother to protect them. They are secure. They know where their food comes from. They haven't seen life at its broadest. They haven't seen death. I had seen death and I knew what could happen.

I've never really got over the fear of swallowing. Even the other day I was ready for hospital, simply because I couldn't eat. It's getting worse now I'm getting older.

Every day
In what other ways does OCD affect your life?

Your mind is never quiet. It is never relaxed. You're giving yourself all the wrong messages. 'You're stupid. You're an idiot. People don't like you.' Over a period of time this gets worse. It's like an infection or something festering. And like an infection, if you don't get it treated, it just gets worse and worse and worse – until it becomes gangrenous.

Could you describe a typical day?

I wake up and my mind is going over and over with the fear that I'm going to do something foolish or bad. Every day. *Every* day. Over and over. Some people might call it schizophrenia, but it's not. I'm not hearing *other* voices, I'm hearing my own. During the day, my mind is never free. I'm always ruminating. I'm going over and over in my mind how I feel. It affects my work, my concentration, I am forgetful, I make mistakes and then I start to be indecisive. I can no longer make the decisions that everyone else makes. I have constant doubt. I can't decide to go out, because if I do, I may *do* something. I may steal something. I may make a fool of myself. There are times I have the feeling that I may shout out loud. If I'm in a cinema, I fear that I might lose control. I fear that I will go down to the casino and gamble all my money away. Shopping is a dreadful thing. The crowds. I'm afraid I'm going to touch somebody.

Last weekend I went to an air show interstate, and I kept thinking I was going to touch a particular woman inappropriately. I kept thinking about it and thinking about it and thinking about it and thinking about it. Another person with OCD might go to the air show and they couldn't eat the food or drink the water. In my case it is a guilt thing, but for other people with OCD it may be germ thing. They may wash their hands once, and then they may wash them again, and again, and again. They may fear touching envelopes, or food, or other people. It's all about fear and worry. It's just constant flight.

Have you ever done inappropriate things?
No.

How has OCD affected your relationship with the people around you?

When I first had my brain disturbance I looked at other people in a distorted way. My feelings towards them changed for the worse. I couldn't make eye contact with people any more. I didn't see the goodness in them. When I was younger if I saw a disabled child or someone in trouble I was always helpful, but after the disturbance I saw them as being weak. Perhaps I recognised their weakness in myself. I was so self-conscious around them.

At home, if you see that the people around you are

happy it doesn't seem quite right, because *you* aren't happy. I know it's irrational, but that's the way it is. And then you start to pick at them. Gnaw at them. And then in some cases you try to change them to the way *you* want them to be. You expect them to do things the way you want. You expect them to clean the house more often. Your meals have to be dead on time. You want them to wear certain clothes because you feel that what they're wearing is not right. You don't like the way their hair is.

It happens at work too. If your workmates don't think the way you do, you try to get them to agree with you. And in the end they disown you and think that you're odd, and that's fair enough. We become very self-centred. Very selfish. My father was a very selfish man. He expected favours to be done for him, but if you asked him to do you a favour, he wouldn't do it. I can see that that way of treating people is not right. And I'm learning to do it differently . . . things have changed . . .

What has brought about that change?

I'm out of a stressful environment. The best times now are when I sit down quietly and put things into perspective. I have the time to reflect . . . that I didn't steal anything from the shops in the morning for instance . . . that I haven't done anything wrong. It's quiet. When I was at work I could never stop.

The whole equation

Over the years I've noticed that people with OCD are very sensitive people. We let things hurt us very easily. It is as though we are too finely tuned. It is as though we are looking for the reasons that we shouldn't be looking for. Why are we here? What are we doing here? Life should be lived to the fullest, but the OCD people just take it too seriously. It's better to be involved . . . with your wife, with your garden, with your social club . . . and I believe there is a genetic factor there as well . . . I believe my aunt and my mother both had it.

Do you see a connection between that genetic factor and the traumatic events you recounted?

I think that OCD can lie dormant in people, and then it just needs that little bit extra to push you over the edge – to push that gene into action. It's a combination of genes and of events in one's life. It's like the soldier in a war, who can cope with only so much. It depends on how much we can tolerate.

And I think it may also have something to do with a chemical reaction in the brain. Everything we do is a chemical reaction in the brain and when we have a trauma or something like that, we have a reaction in the brain that stops our bodies from functioning in the normal way. The normal way is to face fear head on. In the brain of the OCD person we have to unblock the part of the brain where the fear is locked. I'm not talking about sticking a probe in. I'm talking about emotionally unblocking it. We've got to let it out. But I also think that in my case there is some sort of weakness in my brain and the things that happened in my childhood simply brought that out.

I once saw a doctor who said that I had a very weak central nervous system, because I'm also very sensitive to drugs. So that is another theory.

Sometimes I also wonder whether it might be a sort of post-traumatic stress disorder, that was passed on to me through my mother, because she was pregnant with me during the bombings in the war. But behaviour is also part of it. My mother's anxious behaviour might have passed on to me.

Another thing I'd like to point out is that doctors have never asked, 'What do you do as an occupation, George?' They've never thought to give me a blood test or an allergy test. They never asked me what I've been handling or what I've come into contact with. At work I was handling metals and solvents and oils. Cyanide. I would like doctors to treat people with OCD the same as everybody else – give them blood tests, look at the whole equation. They should take *everything* into account. I think it's a bit like a big jigsaw.

But still I wish to stress that the most important thing is for people to have OCD treated *early*, so that it doesn't become entrenched in one's life. Those treatments weren't available when I was young.

What treatments are available now?

They've recognised a gene and they also have SSRIs that control chemicals in the brain and provide relief from the continual trauma of the rumination. Therapy is also important. Locking people in mental institutions, feeding them with drugs and not having a proper therapy is a no-no to me. I've been into the hospital and there really was no therapy there. And that's wrong. It's wrong to just let people wander around. People should be *doing* things. I do a lot of computing now and that's good because it takes my mind off everything. Drugs are just a support. You *must be helped to change your way of thinking*. You can't rely solely on the drugs. You must have inter-action. You must have therapy. You must have someone to *guide* you so that you can live a life of quality.

And I'd like to say that kindness and understanding are so important too and they are so often lacking in psychiatric care. They help your self-esteem, your confidence. You go to a doctor's surgery and all they do is look at the time, bring out the prescription pad, sign the prescription and then out you go. If you get a caring doctor, a caring nurse, a caring social worker it is everything. Kindness. *Compassion!* My GP right now is quite good. He sees a lot of people with OCD. My psychiatrist is not a bad fellow but he doesn't do any therapy with me. He just asks me what I've been doing. I can see that I'm becoming more of a friend to him and I don't want that. I want him to talk to me more about my specific problems rather than talk to me about computing or everyday things. I want a doctor who treats me as a patient. I know I'm going to have to change psychiatrists.

I used to attend GROW, which is a government-funded self-help organisation. It taught me a lot of wisdom. It taught me that God doesn't make rubbish. It taught me that no matter how you feel, you're still a good person. It taught me that the way you *think* is not always right – that it's important to stay in touch with reality, not to isolate yourself and to do things that are normal and natural, things that everybody else does. And GROW was good because of the interaction with others – knowing that you're not the only one with mental or emotional problems. I went to GROW for over twenty years and I think that helped me more than the psychiatrists.

So overall the medical framework hasn't really helped you?

Well in my case the OCD is chronic. It is like being a diabetic. A diabetic doesn't get better. With mental illness, I can get relief, but my doctor told me that there is no cure and I simply have to manage it. That's why I don't think there should be any stigma. People feel that they are odd. They fear what people will say about them. I think it stops many people from getting proper treatment.

Could you give an example of that stigmatisation from your own life?

I went interstate by train last weekend for that air show. I mentioned to three ladies I was talking to that I had an 'anxiety disorder' and one woman said to me, 'You don't *look* sick.' And I thought, 'Well, *what* is sick?' There are so many people with diabetes, heart complaints or asthma who don't look sick. It is a silly thing to say to someone, because they're really saying, 'Well you're *acting* normally!' They associate mental illness with someone who is stupid and acts like an idiot! Winston Churchill had very bad bipolar disorder and he brought England through the Second World War. Napoleon had schizophrenia. Many of the great people in our world today suffer from all kinds of things! Where is the point of normal? The main point I think is that if the sufferer is in *pain*, well then you've got to try to sort that out.

But the fact is that some people live with OCD and they don't really know they've got it, because they accept it as a norm and aren't suffering. They might just live with a very strict code of cleanliness or expect a lot from their children.

Lots of children might even have OCD, and it might start to show itself when they hide in their rooms, when they don't want to eat with the rest of the family or when they spend a lot of time in the toilet or the bathroom.

It's important that people are *educated* about the fact that these illnesses exist, so that they can go and see someone about it. It is so vital to recognise it, and this is where the stigma must be addressed. If you see a child having difficulty breathing, you quickly realise that it's not normal, and you immediately take them to the doctor, so that they might diagnose asthma, for instance.

And then the child may be given medication and some sort of therapy for breathing control. What's the difference between *that* and a mental problem? You can get medication, counselling, therapy . . .

There's been a lot in the media addressing the stigma associated with depression. Politicians readily admit that they suffer from depression. People are beginning to understand it. I don't think there's much said about OCD. I've heard from doctors that along with depression, OCD could well become an epidemic in a few years.

What do you put that down to?

The media. The continual watching of violence on the TV. The anxiety of 'you've got to have this, you've got to have that, you've got to be good looking, you can't be fat'. People tend to overlook the *good* things about themselves.

We are human beings. We are *unique*. We are *special*. It's our soul. We each have our own unique psyche. Our own unique way of doing things. A robot, a mechanical thing, doesn't have that uniqueness. It is so important that we feel good with ourselves no matter whether we are mentally retarded, mentally ill, blind or whatever. A criminal can even feel good about themselves! We need *love* for one another. We need to be accepted for who we are. I don't feel good with myself but I can see that that's the way to go. From the time I had that thought about killing my mother, I felt like a bad person. It was so traumatic, disturbing, terrible . . . and I have lived with it for so long.

How do you envisage the future?

I don't want to live long.

Who wants to live like this? I don't have a quality of life. It's not the quantity that's the thing, it's the *quality*.

If tomorrow someone said to me, 'For the next ten

years you're going to have a lovely life, you won't have much money, but you'll be *you*! You'll be *George* again. You'll be content within yourself and with other people. You'll have your self-esteem back again. Would you prefer that ten-year life I just described or would you like live for another twenty years and stay as you are?'

. . . well, I'd pick the ten-year option.

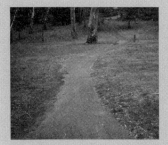

Sarah

Sarah is 33 years old. She has been diagnosed with dissociative identity disorder and atypical schizophrenia. As a child she was severely ritually abused by a satanic cult. *'I don't think we ever achieve the ultimate, but aiming towards the ultimate brings us closer to it. This photo is like the path or journey towards that ultimate.'*

I have a quote that I made up for myself:

> The journey of life will take you many places but wherever you are, there you will be.

The journey of my life is pretty rocky. There are lots of different experiences. Sometimes there are positive things and sometimes there are difficult things. It's like the winding road of a real journey. When you're going on a real journey you pass through different kinds of scenery. Sometimes there's just one long hard road with no scenery and no stops. Other times there might be a town with more variety, more trees and more green hills around.

But along the way you might also break down. You either have to learn to fix things yourself by using your own skills or you might need to call someone in to help you. Knowing what you can handle and when you need help is part of being on the journey. It's also part of the journey to know when you're running on empty and you have to find somewhere to fill up.

My experience of the journey is that I can see the scenery but I'm still travelling through. The scenery is still under the cover of disaster and pain from my past. It's not yet where my life is. The green and the interesting things are there to help me along the way and to help me move on. The road is still a long road . . . like over the Hay Plain in NSW . . . there aren't many stops for petrol . . .

What does that metaphor bring to your life?

It's about coming to a sense of peace, of understanding and of accepting my life wherever I'm at and wherever it takes me. If I deal with what I have at that time in the best way I possibly can, with the resources that are around me or with the resources that I have within, then I'll continue on the journey.

What do you mean when you say, 'continue on the journey'?

That I won't give up.

I suppose trying to stay alive has been a pretty big thing for me . . . or rather, trying not to die. As far as being suicidal goes, I don't necessarily want to die, but I'm not all that keen on living either. It's not that I particularly want death, it's more that I want to stop the suffering and get out of the pain. Day after day. Year after year. It gets overwhelming and then I don't know what to do with myself. Sometimes I just can't see a way out. I just can't handle it . . . but I've *had* to handle it . . . and I've *decided* to handle it. That decision doesn't stop me from *feeling* suicidal but it stops me from actually doing anything about it.

How did you get to the point of deciding that you would live?

I've often wondered that myself!

If I think about suicide, I think about the consequences.

I don't know what would happen if I died. I don't know what the afterlife experiences would be like. It's a bit like the devil you know is better than the devil you don't. At other times I think I've come too far to ruin all my hard work. If I cut my life short I won't ever be able to achieve what I think is possible. Sometimes I just hold on to whatever I can to stay alive.

But knowing I won't commit suicide has sometimes been frustrating, because when you get to a point at which you feel you can't keep going, it would be easier in that moment to be able to end it.

What do you do now when you feel suicidal?

If it gets really bad I go to the emergency department of a hospital. But I also might ring a friend and say I'm feeling suicidal. I try to get away from saying I will kill myself, because it doesn't sit comfortably with me any more, especially with a particular close friend that I have . . . she allows me to really face it . . . that helps me get a bit of a break.

What does she do to allow that to happen?

She says that she wouldn't want me to kill myself but that she would understand if I did. She walks alongside me. She is *with* me on the same level, she is equal and that makes an enormous difference. She also knows how deep things have been for me. She understands . . . and I can talk about how I'm feeling, which is not easy for me, because I've had *so* much rejection and *so* much of 'you-have-to-be-this-way-you-have-to-be-that-way'.

The other day when I was with my therapist I cried in her office for the first time in about two-and-a-half years. In the past I felt she wouldn't have accepted or liked me if I showed her how I was feeling. Showing people how I feel has been a *huge* thing . . . I've always thought it was bad or that it was wrong. Showing how I feel has meant rejection for me, it has meant isolation . . . and it's isolation, for whatever reason, that can lead to depression, and then a further downward spiral into suicidal feelings. So breaking isolation, breaking through the barriers of someone who is feeling hopeless is *so* important.

Showing how I feel has also meant having no friends. Because everything is so intense with me, people don't know how to deal with my feelings on a friendship level . . . my life just doesn't go there . . .

What do you think makes it hard for people?

I think the biggest thing that other people find difficult is their fear. Fear of pain. Fear of death. Fear of intense situations. Fear can make someone either fight or take flight . . . the 'fight or flight' stuff. So people either lecture you and tell you what you should or shouldn't do with your life, or they back off completely. My friend never runs away from it but she doesn't push me into things either. She sticks by me. She's not afraid of the difficulties. She can see my qualities and the positives in my life and she wants to help me achieve those.

But I think it's also fear of other things. People fear that their time and energy are being used. They fear that the person in need may become dependent on them. People are comfortable in their own lives and they don't want that disturbed. If you're dealing with people like me you have to set strong boundaries and guidelines and people just don't have those kinds of skills.

My attitude at the moment is that it takes a special person to put up with me, to be able to stick with me through the difficulties, to be able to support me when I need support . . . to allow everything to come out.

Is your friend able to set strong boundaries and guidelines?

Yeah . . . like . . . You can talk to me any time but I'll let you know if I'm available or not. It's okay for you to ring me but it's okay for me to say no. Or, it's okay for you to want support, I'll give you support, but sometimes I won't be there for you.

And you're okay with those?

Yeah. I've come to accept them. Knowing those boundaries has helped me know where I stand and where she stands, when I am going too far or how far I can go. And they're not manipulative. They're not controlling. The support that this friend gives me is really helping me. It's understanding, it's empathetic . . . I know she's genuine.

The fact is, if you've only got one person supporting you and she's the only person you can talk to and have personal contact with apart from your therapist, then it *can* become a burden. If there were more people and a system in place there would be less pressure for everyone. People are afraid that when you build up systems in order to try to help people like me, that we would become more and more burdensome . . . but we wouldn't. It would become easier for the people giving support and also for the people needing support. It would be more of a team effort. And the boundaries could be set from the very beginning. I wish to add that someone who really wants to get better and improve their life is always extremely appreciative of any help they receive.

I'd just like to say that I've got a theory about suicide as well . . . It's that people who love life the most, are the most suicidal.

How does that apply in your own life?

I think suicide is an enormous conflict between life and between pain and suffering . . . between seeing what's out there but not knowing how to access it . . . it's about wanting more out of life. It's what you *don't* have rather than what you *do* have.

I have had intensely good experiences and real positives in my life – and I experienced them to the full – but when I have the difficult experiences, my ability to access those good experiences seems blocked. It's about trying to achieve a better life and satisfaction on the journey . . . because I *know* that it's out there, I *know* that it's possible, I *know* that I'm capable of it . . . I can see that other people *do* have positive experiences and achieve milestones in their lives. But there are times when it just feels as though it's all too hard. The emotional pain of that conflict of feeling, time and time again, makes me feel I can't take it any more.

I have spent a lot of time in my life observing because I never had friends or role models . . . I looked at other people's lives and tried to copy them. I tried to copy the good things or the positive things that I would like in myself. I know that sounds like I'm really unwell but that's how I've lived to be where I am. I see what I like in people and I basically copy that. I also see what I don't like, and say, 'I never want to be like that.' I wonder why everyone can't do that. Why do they say they don't like things? Why can't people just change? Be like this or be like that? That's how I've lived.

But I suppose the danger is that you lose your sense of self.

How would you describe your sense of self?

I probably don't have a very good sense of who I am. I can identify with things on the outside but when it comes to identifying things within, I stumble. I pick up things from my environment and I make them part of myself, rather than initiating or identifying who I really am. I can see the way people see me or the way people think I am, but I don't *feel* that. I feel like I'm just doing things because that's what people want. I feel like I'm just performing.

Where did that sense of having to perform come from?

It came from the sense of not being accepted. Of isolation. Of rejection. Of being bullied by kids at school. Of not fitting in but wanting to fit in. Of being alone but not wanting to be alone. Things like that . . . so you just make yourself into a person or a character that people can accept . . .. But it's all really difficult because you can't hide forever. You can't be one way when you're really not that way. If people saw the real me or really knew what I was like they wouldn't like me. That's pretty much what I go by.

But the mental health system can also take away a person's sense of self. They use the medical model, which focuses on a person's pathology. When you focus on a condition or one small set of circumstances in a person's life called mental illness, a person's identity can become *that*. People can start to believe the label and identity they are given and believe that they are not as capable as the next person; they take on the associated stigma. Other people see the label and don't see the real person behind it.

Trying to get through that barrier to the real person and then developing the real person rather than developing the condition is something society and the mental health system doesn't really understand.

Some people who are given a diagnosis or a label experience relief. Do you think that this relief might be tied to the provision of some sense of identity?

I've experienced that relief myself. If I don't know what I'm dealing with, if I don't have a name for something, then it's harder to work on it. It's like I'm searching but I'm in mid-air or in limbo.

I see the diagnosis as a *tool* on the journey . . . it's a tool to fix a breakdown if I need to. When people think of labels, they either throw the baby out with the bath-water and believe people shouldn't have any labels at all or believe them wholeheartedly and believe that they're the only thing in a person's life. I think labels are okay, it's just the way they're *used* that is the problem. If the box becomes all of who you are then that's damaging. My life is bigger than the label.

But at the moment, there *is* a shift in the mental health system to the recovery model. I don't like the use of the word 'model' because it implies another set of guidelines and another box, but it's a start. It's more about a recovery attitude that focuses on a person holistically: a person's life, what they're experiencing and how they relate to the world and people. I think a person's sense of identity can only come about in relation to their society. If they feel comfortable in their space, in their world and within their interpersonal relationships, they can begin to build on the positives in their lives. They can build on their gifts and talents and so build up their sense of self. It's important that people find out who they really are. If we can't be who we are then that's a constant grief process.

What else do you feel the mental health system could offer people beyond the model you mentioned?

Psychotherapy rather than pharmacotherapy. Symptoms need to be treated on a therapeutic basis rather than a medical one. People need to talk, be accepted and understood. People need to be able to understand their *own* condition and their *own* lives rather than have questions directed at them about what professional people need to know.

A good step forward has been the implementation of mental health key workers. My mental health key worker has been really helpful and supportive in my life, helping me achieve goals and encouraging me in things I have been successful with. She has been practical and encouraging.

But it's my private therapist who has been really important. Her understanding and knowledge of multiple personality disorder has been really vital. She's guided me through. She's really different to anyone else I have experienced, particularly in the mental health system.

How is she different?

She's hasn't focused on my diagnosis. She's focused on my own experience and my ability to share it. She has allowed me to get stronger through talking and through support. She hasn't been trying to gain information to understand my situation in *her* mind, she's helping me to understand and come to terms with my situation in my *own* mind. I've also been able to completely trust her and so that's helped me to trust myself and my own memories and experiences. I don't think she works to any particular model either. I think she uses whatever is right for a person and a situation at any particular time.

At the beginning of the interview you spoke about your experiences in terms of the winding road of a journey. Where are you on that journey at present?

I was coasting pretty well for a while and then things started to flare up again really badly. But even when I was coasting I was still overcoming difficulties, overcoming amotivation, overcoming disorganisation in my thinking and my life. My life never feels organised. So even when I was going okay, there were still issues. And then all of a sudden things just flared up again. Issues started coming back that I thought I'd dealt with. I'm tired. I'm worn out. I can't keep doing this. How can I live like this? I still want to do things. I'm still capable of doing things. But my health, my situation, my feelings take over.

What sorts of issues have resurfaced?

Mainly memories from the past. Reliving experiences. It's a pretty grey area as far as mental health goes. But things like torture and mind control . . . that sort of thing . . . its memories but also programming that my therapist and other people have helped me identify. The further I get on my journey, the more I start to succeed in something, the harder I fall and the harder I have to try in order to get back on track again. It's not just a mindset of conditioning. There are deeper and stronger things involved that are pretty much out of my control. That's what started coming up again. And that affects my disorganisation, my routines, my schizophrenia . . .

You spoke of your experiences as a grey area with regard to mental health. What did you mean by that?

The grey area is not with regard to schizophrenia. It's with regard to the abuse and the dissociative identity disorder (DID) diagnosis. They aren't really recognised or understood. A lot of time has been spent researching schizophrenia, bipolar and other mental illness, but with DID, the research and the understanding is minimal.

How do *you* understand DID?

I'm still coming to an understanding of it. DID covers the spectrum from general everyday dissociation to multiple personality disorder. Everyday dissociation is just distancing. It's like highway hypnosis . . . when you're going on a long journey and you're doing all the right things like driving the car, watching the road, watching for other cars, but you lose all sense of time and everything else. Multiple personality disorder is a complete split from the host personality to another personality. People have amnesic periods or memory loss or complete change of character, complete change of voice and even eye colour, body temperature, even male/female, clothes, interests, talents. One personality might be really good at playing the piano while another might not have a clue how to do it, even though it's within the same body.

How are you affected by DID?

My DID consists of personalities but it doesn't consist of complete amnesia. I believe I've somehow developed a really good system of memory and communication due to obsessive thinking. I continually go over things in my mind or continually replay situations obsessively rather than forgetting them. 'Should I do this?' 'Should I do that?' 'Did I say the right thing?'

So it's like a system of continuity that remains through everything.

Yeah. But it's not a continuity of feeling and it's not a continuity of experience. At one moment I can feel that everything's great and everything's okay and that I'm well, but the next moment I feel completely messed up and I can't cope any more, even with getting through the day. Consistency of feeling in a situation or consistency of experience isn't there. Consistency of memory isn't always there either. Sometimes it takes me a while to remember things . . . I might have to go through my mind to find a memory of what happened, but it doesn't constitute a complete break in memory. Personalities are strong but they're not *so* split off from me or not *so* dissociated that I have amnesia. They are distinct but they won't come across as being really distinct to someone who doesn't know me.

When you speak of feeling great one day and then completely messed up the next, are you talking of two distinct personalities?

I believe so. Right now I wouldn't be able to say who is talking, but in therapy I can because there is an element of trust and an element of consistency that enables it to come out. It would be good for me to identify who's who and what's what at any particular time so that I could work on it. At least I might be able to understand myself even if other people don't.

But the fact is that in my day-to-day life I have to try to *be* consistent, I have to try to present in certain ways so that people will accept me and understand me and not be confused by the way I'm acting or the way I'm talking. It's probably part of the cover-up . . . but I also manage to cover up for myself as well.

Do you think people get confused by the way you act and talk?

Not by the way I present at any one time. Over a period of time people may get confused. They don't necessarily know they're confused, they just back off and don't get involved. They feel uncomfortable. An acquaintance who doesn't know I have DID once left a message on my answering machine that said, 'It's good to hear your message, because you always sound the same on it.' She didn't realise what she was saying!

You spoke of lack of continuity in your experience or your feelings. Could you describe this a little more?

I might start a course at TAFE or uni. The first time I go there it's really good and I participate in everything. The next week my experience has completely changed and I've lost the experience I had. I know I'm capable of doing the course but I have two completely different experiences of it. But I still have to participate because I don't want to let myself or others down. I have to keep my life together. I try to go back to my initial experience and create an outer stability because I can't find any inner stability. It's a lot like having to perform and so it becomes a lot more pressurised. As a result I end up stuck with all this stuff that I am interested in and capable of doing, but am unable to cope with.

Another thing that is related to the DID is having different points of view on the same issue. I see different sides . . . the positive and the negative. I don't feel safe in any point of view. I don't feel safe in things I say. If I say something positive then it has been challenged. If I say something negative then that has been challenged too.

By whom?

I was ritually abused by a satanic cult . . . But I'm hesitant to use the word 'cult' because it can describe many different organisations with many different ways of operating. Satanic cults are very underground and secretive, and they practise ritual abuse and torture. I would also like to point out that I wasn't *in* that cult or *part* of that cult; I was severely ritually abused *by* that cult. It was never my choice. It was simply part of growing up. It was part of a very unstable situation. Things were twisted; things were taken away and then given back to me, back to front . . . if I was happy I was told off, if I was having a hard time I was told to pick myself up . . . I was always trying to find a point of stability . . .

When you're talking with me now, you have some quite concrete points of view. How have you come to those?

I've worked very hard to make sense of the world and make sense of myself. I've tried very hard to make something concrete and stable out of something that feels very unstable and unreal. I've had to put words to things that seem very hard to understand. I have to fit into society so I work extra hard and put a lot of energy into saying things that make sense. It's so important to me that people understand what I'm saying, because if they don't, it means rejection, isolation and misunderstanding. I've often said that mental illness is like speaking a different language. You're just not able to fit in with the rules of society and the way people generally communicate.

If I do have to say something or have an opinion, I try to work out the pros and cons and then come to a conclusion. Sometimes when I'm talking I can be quite slow because I'm working so hard at it. Sometimes I think what I'm saying can sound confused or doesn't make sense but people still say, 'Yeah, but it does make sense.'

Having spoken about DID, what is the relationship between it and schizophrenia?

It's pretty complicated . . . they *are* polarised as far as being two different disorders. I only see a relationship through the abuse. I believe they were created from the same type of abuse . . . satanic ritual abuse (SRA) . . . stress creates one and stress creates the other.

You can't have DID without having been through some sort of abuse as a child. People simply don't split off under normal circumstances. It only happens under extraordinary trauma or difficult circumstances that the child can't handle on its own.

In people who have a predisposition to schizophrenia there is usually a trauma that triggers it off. It can be any type of trauma: a breakdown in relationships, being sacked at a job . . .

How does schizophrenia manifest in you?

The positive symptoms of schizophrenia are when people hear voices, have hallucinations, delusions . . .

those things are 'out there'. I have the negative symptoms of schizophrenia. They take away from who you are: amotivation, disorganised thinking, lack of enjoyment, lack of satisfaction, inability to connect to things. That's why it's so difficult, because it's not the usual symptoms. They don't stop me from *wanting* to experience things or knowing that I *can* do them, they just stop me from actually experiencing it.

My therapist and I think I had schizophrenia in primary school and it was most likely triggered off by the abuse.

Do you remember feeling different at school?

Yeah a lot. And very traumatised in school by peers and also by my home situation. But I don't remember a great deal of my home situation. I do remember that from a very young age I never wanted to be there. I wished someone would take me out of my home to live with another family. That's an indication to me that something severely wrong was happening at the time. I realise now that some family members were in a cult that we don't know all the specific details of yet.

We?

Me and the therapist I'm working with. But it's actually a bit ambiguous when I say 'we'. When people say 'we', it's usually a strong sign that they have other personalities. I try to avoid it so people can't pick up on my personalities. I try to avoid saying 'we' or 'I' or anything. I just say things like, 'It hasn't been picked up on' or something like that.

Do you have any memories of that abuse?

I'm getting memories of it now, but I don't know what memory is. I reckon that's a blocking mechanism.

What is memory to *you* then?

I would define memories for most people, as getting pictures, with clear details and clear understanding, like watching a video or movie of something that's happening. But that's not what memories always consist of. Sometimes it will be more of an experiential thing, a symptom thing . . .

Could you give me an example?

Yeah. Being locked up in a coffin and buried.

So that's not on a video screen in your head but comes as a bodily sense?

A body memory. It's a knowing that it happened. And a feeling of everything associated with that. I suppose a lot of people would easily deny that sort of thing, but I've come to a situation where I have to accept it to be able to move on. If I don't accept it, it just gets more and more traumatic. If I work through the memories, if I work through the situation, and talk about it and relive it . . . which I don't relive but it happens . . . I don't *do* it but . . .

Are you saying that although you're reliving it, there's actually no conscious input from you to relive it?

Yeah. Yeah. So when I start reliving a memory it comes as trauma. At the moment I'm going through memories of being in a coffin, buried. In the past I wouldn't have been able to identify that as a memory, it would have been just one big ball of trauma. I would not have been able to specify what was happening and why it was happening. But now things are starting to separate out. I can say, 'This is what I am going through.'

What effect has being able to separate it out, had on your life?

It has allowed me not to dissociate from the trauma, but to stand back and say, 'This is what is happening.' It's not that it makes it any easier, but it gives me some distance to be able to think it through. It allows me to see why I'm feeling like I'm feeling. It allows me to put it into some context, rather than have it completely over-take my mind. It's also allowing me to realise that the trauma is not *all* my life . . . that I do have a life . . . that I can live and function with the abilities and qualities that I do have. The trauma is something that's added on to that, which makes things very difficult for me some-times, but it doesn't mean that I can't do it. Sometimes I just have to adjust the way I do things, or take time out, or deal with the situation.

I needed . . . probably not today, but yesterday . . . the mental health system doesn't cater for these issues very well because they are more of an acute-based system. As I said earlier, they deal with the symptoms rather than deal with the problem. They don't understand that I'm not just being psychotic and that you can't just give me medication and that will be it. Their treatment doesn't fit my situation. To get through it I have to work with different personalities, communications and relationships. Anyone who has been through any kind of abuse has those kinds of issues, but mine are probably amplified because of the severity of what happened. It makes it even harder.

What was it that you needed from the mental health system yesterday?

I needed a place to go . . . not to hospital, not be assessed, not be interviewed, and not be treated medi-cally. There *are* places around. Here in NSW there's a place called Mayumarri[8] which is an Aboriginal name.

---

8 Mayumarri runs affordable healing centres for people who have experienced childhood trauma. They have centres in NSW, Queensland, Victoria and Western Australia (with plans for one in England and one in Tasmania). National Information Line is 1300 760 580 and website is www.mayumarri.com.au

They have a week-long program for people who are going through experiences of any type of child abuse. I've been there a few times, and it has really helped me. I need specific counselling to deal with the personalities and to deal with the abuse. I need to understand the times and dates and triggers that cults use to actively and psychically work on people to bring them down or call them back to the cult.

Do you feel that this is still happening to you?

Yeah. And I need somewhere where I can deal with it that is separate from the rest of my life, rather than struggle through and wear myself down even more.

I know of someone who actually committed suicide. She was getting callbacks. Another personality would become active, a very strong male, and she would catch the train to a specific area where the cult was, so that they could torture her. People tried to stop her, but she was so strong that they couldn't.

She was also cutting up and self-harming and even hospitals wouldn't take her. Some of the personalities were programmed to self-harm and there was one personality that was programmed to harm people who tried to help her. At one time someone was trying to help her and she tried to choke them. She was so aggressive and strong. But people probably did the wrong thing with her, because the condition was even less understood then.

Why do you feel they did the wrong thing?

It was the way she was being treated. They were misguided. They were trying to call out the personalities and cast them away in a similar manner to demons. They were trying to heal through prayer and deliverance, but in the cult, programming was in the name of Satan and was used against Christianity and against God. All kinds of Christian symbols are used in their rituals so that anything to do with Christianity can be a trigger. Some personalities would freak out if even the name of God or Christian symbols like crosses were used. It can be retraumatising for the personalities. She was getting retraumatised so she was cutting up even more. Her situation was misunderstood.

There's a book called *First Person Plural* by Dr Cameron West. It's about DID but not SRA. It's about sexual abuse and DID. The author was trying to force himself not to notice his personalities and he actually ended up cutting himself more. It got to a stage where he was told that he had to face the personalities otherwise he would keep getting worse. In America they actually have hospitals that are DID specific, so they videotaped him when he was switching personalities and then replayed it so that he could see what was happening. In the end he spent time with his personalities. He read them books, kids' stories, drew pictures . . . and he started to improve. That's how I see the situation with that person I described. The retraumatisation just makes things worse. It makes the personalities act out more. With the right kind of treatment, they're responsive . . . just like a little child. Although my personalities manifest a bit differently, I've also found these issues true in my own life.

You mentioned that you were also getting callbacks. What do you believe their purpose is in your life?

I believe it's to ruin my life, so that I end up in gaol, or dead. I felt that very strongly the other day . . . I *sense* that. I tend to start something, get really good at it, feel successful and then I crash and become unwell. I either have to stop working or I end up in hospital for short periods of time, not functioning, traumatised and feeling suicidal. I realise now that this is part of the callback or trigger. But this time I've managed to keep working and keep all my appointments. I've tried really hard to hold on to my job and everything I'm doing. My friend has helped a lot but it's also through sheer determination to get through.

When you were hospitalised, what was your experience there?

It's different to a lot of other people's experiences. Hospital has actually been an escape for me. If I could have lived in hospital I would have. As a child I never actually lived in an institution, but with the cult and the abuse I had no freedom and no choice. I was institutionalised without being institutionalised. I wasn't allowed to watch TV, I wasn't allowed to use the phone, I wasn't allowed to make friends, choose what I ate, choose what I wore. I think hospital was a way of continuing that, because I didn't have to make my own choices or make my own decisions. When I am suicidal, unable to cope or traumatised, I present myself to hospital and say I need to be there. Then I have some routine back. Going to hospital has mainly been a safety valve when I can't cope but it isn't an ideal alternative, because it isn't necessarily therapeutic and doesn't always help you move on.

You mentioned Mayumarri as an alternative to hospital.

I feel something like that would be really valuable not only for people who have experienced child abuse but also for people who have experienced SRA. So it might be SRA specific and DID specific.

You were saying that Mayumarri has a non-medical approach.

They have a knowledge and understanding of human relationships, healing and recovery that the mental health system doesn't always understand. The system only reinforces isolation; it only treats the *symptoms* of depression, of being suicidal or of trauma. For instance it treats post-traumatic stress disorder as a *disorder* rather than a condition of humanity.

So rather than a disorder, you see it as a valid reaction to circumstances?

Yeah. Yeah. Someone said to me the other day, 'Crying is good. It's a normal reaction.' And I said, 'Yeah, but it's a normal reaction to horrible experiences.' How can you call crying good, when you have to cry in the first place? It might be healing and it might help you get through something but the reason why it's there *isn't* good.

What did your time at Mayumarri give you?

Inner strength in dealing with the inner child. Healing the wounded child within me. Giving the inner child the time and attention that it never had as a child. It's what it's screaming out for . . . the inner child is like the abused part of the adult.

It's also about experiencing the emotions and feelings instead of blocking everything inside. It's important to bring things out into the open and not keep secrets . . . even from myself. Doing that is cathartic, it's releasing, it's healing. It's not very easy and I don't think I do it very well but it does go a long way towards being able to understand and relate to my own life.

Mayumarri also has routines but not strict ones . . . it's not like you *have* to do this or that. It's more that routine is helpful. It's about doing activities like working around the property that are outside of what you're feeling and outside of your own experiences. It's also about relationship . . . it's about doing things together.

You've brought up relationship a number of times in a number of different ways. What is important about relationship for you?

I believe that people need relationships to function in the world, but because of the severe isolation in my childhood I didn't know how to relate. That's why people like me might be called dysfunctional, because I've had a breakdown in relationships. Relationships are very important to me because I need to be able to express myself.

In the past I would lose a lot of my energy being with people . . . it was draining. Most of my life I have only dealt with adults, even in primary school. It's always been teachers or professionals, never peers, never people that I could just talk to for the sake of talking to. That's a grief I have.

Do you find it less draining to be with people now?

Yeah. Yeah I do. It actually gives me more energy than being on my own. If I do something with someone else I can do it fairly well, but if I do it on my own it's like I'm pushing uphill.

How has that change come about?

Therapy. Working on issues and starting to understand the world around me. And probably medication as well. Medication has probably changed the schizophrenia side of things – the way I relate to the world, my energy. People have noticed that I'm getting positive experiences out of doing things rather than being drained by doing them.

So medication is helpful for you?

This one more than any other I've been on. It's an atypical anti-psychotic that targets different parts of the brain to most other anti-psychotics and has fewer side effects.

Apart from the medication you are currently on, what has been your overall impression of the medication that you've been given?

Medication has been helpful and has had a hand in partly stabilising me – 'a difficult thing in a difficult situation'. But it's no quick fix and I've found the side effects pretty terrible . . . weight gain and my whole body is just completely packing up. I feel like an old lady sometimes, in my movement, in aches and pains. I used to be really fit and really active, but now I feel I've lost all of that. I think if I hadn't been on medication I would still have been able to play some kind of sport . . . but I'm trying to get back to it. I think I've lost some things, but that doesn't mean I can't do something if I want to.

How do you envisage the future overall?

My main goal in life is to find some sort of emotional and personal stability: to find satisfaction, to feel organised, to feel like I'm coping with things.

Work is very important to me. It's a way of not focusing on my condition and my inabilities but rather focusing on my abilities and focusing on being productive in society. It's not a label of 'being productive in society' but rather it's an experience of receiving and achieving things. A big frustration of experiencing difficulties in your life is not being able to be productive. Our natural selves *are* productive.

Eventually I want a career, full-time work and I want to get paid professionally. Some time ago there was a job advertised in the paper. It didn't require a resume, experience or an interview. So I started with that. I thought that if could stick with that for a year and be consistent at it, it would help me prove that I could do something to another employer. And that's what happened. And now there are things opening up for me in which I can be productive. I feel that whatever little you have, if you don't use it, then you'll lose it. If you start with whatever little you have, then you'll get more.

I think it's important to get out there and do something no matter how you feel. It's like *life* fitness, not physical fitness. With physical fitness you exercise and you get stronger and so you can do more things. I actually feel that my life skills are getting better and that I'm not just a shell any more. I feel more independent and more separate from the world. And that's through practice. It's the journey thing . . . I'm continually pushing through. I'm working on it every day. I'm continually doing what I have to do. Times are still hard but I don't see myself going backwards. I'm getting closer to the top of the mountain.

Joan

Joan is 56 years old . . . *'For me those 56 years have a significance. I first had a breakdown at 27 years of age and it took a further 27 years to undo everything. I was 54 when I drew the triptych below and knew that peace and contentment were now within my life.'*

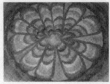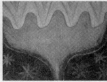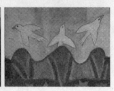

I'd like to start with how I feel now . . .

Most days now, I feel content and at peace with life. Although there are still times when I can feel a little vulnerable, I know I could handle pretty much anything life throws at me.

When I was first asked if there was something I would like from life, it didn't take me too long to work out that there was nothing else to strive for but peace and contentment. There were other smaller goals like a career or a formal education, but the Holy Grail for me was peace and contentment.

Because this peace and contentment is something I came to later in life, I never take it for granted and I doubt I ever will. I had to struggle and fight so very hard to get here and I will cherish it always. In a material sense there is nothing anyone could offer me that would convince me to give it up. I would rather die than give it up.

I believe there are a lot of people out there who do not realise that if they only stood still, they would find the answer within them. It's okay to stop and take stock of your life and work out where you're at. It's okay to take a minute to smell the roses or sit on the beach.

When people speak of striving for something in their lives it is often happiness that comes to mind . . .

People may strive for happiness, but peace and contentment are different from happiness. I certainly experience moments now, when I can sit and be really happy but that happiness is never a full-time thing. It's a passing thing. It's like an elation. Doing this interview, for example, gives me a feeling of happiness because it's out of the ordinary . . . it's special to be sitting here, talking and sharing with you about how it's been for me. Peace and contentment are more subtle than that.

I always knew deep down within, that I had an ability to be contented and at peace, but there was *so* much overshadowing it that I had no idea how to unravel it all; I had no idea how to get this inner person out. It was like a big knot inside, a mixture of confusion, ignorance, terrible feelings of despair, depression, anger and loneliness.

Even when I was very young I was aware of this inner person. Once I understood the concept of leaving home and being free of my mother, I started to wonder, 'Will that be the time I'll be the real me?' But because I'd been so deprived of social knowledge and self-understanding, when I *did* leave home it only added to my burdens. I'd lived in a world of my own up until then and anything remotely getting near that was threatening.

What do you mean by 'world of my own'?

I lived in a fantasy world. It wasn't any particular fantasy. It wasn't like a fairy tale. It was my whole life. My whole being. I didn't cope well in the real world. The real world was an uncaring, cold and heartless world in which older people had all the control. I felt threatened by them and unable to communicate with them. The fantasy world was less painful and more bearable. Although everyday experiences were on the one hand real, I entwined them with my own fantasy. Characters in it were people I knew. They were parent figures I preferred over my own parents. They were nicer than my own. They cared more. I felt they treated me as an individual.

Growing up, at school and as a young adult, I felt alien and ignorant; I felt very different to everyone around me. I didn't understand that I was *me* and that I was unique. It was something I never contemplated. I had always searched for a person with whom I could connect and I had assumed that person would be identical to me. I didn't understand that we are all different and that I wasn't a carbon copy of this person or that person. When I eventually realised that I was unique and that there was no one in the world exactly like me, I started to feel very paranoid and alone.

Could you tell me more about what your childhood was like?

I think the overwhelming thing was, 'Why me?' There were six children and my mother was only abusive to my brother and me. Perhaps we reminded her more of our father than any of the others; he was an alcoholic and abused her physically for fifteen years. When she did leave him, she continued to push the abuse onto us. She'd say: '*Your* father has never paid maintenance for you', '*Your* father . . .' As I come to the end of dealing with it all, there are only two things left: 'Why me?' and the fact that I can't forgive her.

Do you feel that you *should* forgive her?

No. I feel that's God's area. If anyone's going to forgive

her, then He can. I'm not God; I can't play judge and jury and I don't intend to. If she ever *asks* for forgiveness, that would be different. I would consider it. Early in therapy there were occasions when I ended up in hospital just from dealing with various incidents of my childhood. When my sisters heard about them, they'd go back to my mum and ask her, 'Was it true what you did to Joan?' And her reply has always been, 'I don't remember'. To me that's a real denial. If she was going to lie, she'd say she didn't do it. But she never says that.

My mother could never see past herself. She thought she was the centre of the world. I have begun to understand that not one of us is the centre of the world. We might think that as a very young child but then we grow out of it. I don't think my mother ever grew out of it. I think my mother was probably more mentally unstable and unwell than I ever have been, only she had something that I didn't have: she had the ability to domineer and have power over people. I didn't have that. That's probably the only reason that I ended up in hospital so many times and she didn't. When she was domineering and pushing people around, it made her feel good. I didn't have anything in my life to make me feel good.

I know that the issue as to whether children should be taken from their families is a very contentious one, but sometimes I think the damage done by *not* removing children can be very great. That damage can wipe out an individual's potential – for a few years, for half a life, for a whole life. Thinking back over those terribly abusive years, I can remember quite clearly *wanting* desperately to pick up a phone and ask someone to take me out of the family. I remember that *very, very* vividly. It was a time before there was such a thing as a house phone, but I knew where the local public phone was. I *wanted* to go to that phone so very much . . . but I didn't have the initiative.

You mention being hospitalised many times.

At first when I was admitted to hospital they said I'd just had a nervous breakdown. Once I'd been in two or three times, they wanted to diagnose me with something more serious. I was diagnosed with paranoid schizophrenia. Okay. I went along for a few more years and was having different experiences to those that brought about the initial admissions and so they changed it to manic depression (now called bipolar). I'm sure if I experienced something different again, they would come up with something different to call it.

It sounds as though you don't take those diagnoses seriously.

No. They're ridiculous. They fill a space on a form. They help bureaucracy put me somewhere at *one* particular time in my life. That's about all. I feel that I'm a unique person. To me, I am just *me*. If anything, you could probably say that I had an abusive childhood and as a result was traumatised. I grew up living with fear and terror and had no social upbringing, no coping skills and a whole lot of other things.

I don't like the words 'mental illness' either. For large amounts of people, I think the words 'traumatic stress' are more applicable. The fact is that once people actually deal with that traumatic stress, then they no longer have a so-called 'mental illness'. During my years in the mental health service I picked up very clearly that there is a *big* taboo in declaring that your parents played a large part in the creation of your so-called 'mental illness'. I think there is a sense of 'saving face' by calling it an 'illness'. It doesn't put the responsibility on anyone. I think the predisposition to so-called 'mental illness' in a family is directly proportional to how dysfunctional that family is.

I think that labels for people can only ever be really general. Each person within those groups is different and unique. For instance, people with bipolar are meant to have mood swings between the highs and the lows, yet I've had very few highs. I've very rarely been euphoric. Most of the 'illness' has been chronic depression. I've been hospitalised with depression. I also think that when you give people a label, there is no acknowledgment that people are different all the time. Even when people are well, they're always different from day to day. When I go to bed at night I never know how I'm going to be in the morning!

I also think labels can be detrimental, because if at any time I *express* some anger, then it gets written off as illness: 'You're unwell, are you taking your tablets?'

They don't take you seriously?

No. They don't take me seriously. They think I'm overreacting. They can't see that it's normal to express anger from time to time. They probably get just as angry at different times as I do, but for some reason, because they know I have this so-called 'mental illness', they believe that when *I* express anger, it's a sign that I'm getting unwell. And that's *really* unfair. That's almost giving me no right to have an angry feeling.

So there's an expectation that to be 'well' you have to be even-tempered . . .

And that's impossible! I grew up with that. *I grew up with that!* I *know* that you can't go on living like that. They're taking me back to my childhood, during which I wasn't allowed to experience *any* feelings. That's not healthy. We wonder why there is the stigma in the community, and it's because people won't *listen* . . .

I see a difference between listening and hearing. Some people might hear everything but not really *listen* to what you're saying, or to the feeling attached to what you're saying.

Could you go into more detail about that difference?

The difference is that if people listen, then you *know* they're listening by the fact that they understand where you're coming from. Sometimes people might not really understand but still say, 'Oh yeah, yeah . . . I understand.' But you can tell if they don't.

It's a fact that people with a so-called 'mental illness' can tune right in to the person they're communicating with and can usually tell if they're genuine or not. And that is apparently very daunting to a lot of psychiatrists; they're a bit on edge when they talk to us.

Are you saying that you believe people with a so-called 'mental illness' are more sensitive?

Yes. Maybe that is the word. More *sensitive*. More *in tune* with the difference between people hearing what you're saying or *listening* to what you're saying.

As much as the media would have it different we're a group of people that, by and large, are more passive than the general community. If we're more passive then we're saying less and by saying less we're a bit like the wise old owl: we *see* more, we observe.

I've certainly picked up many psychiatrists in the system who are there for all sorts of reasons other than that of really listening to the people they're treating; they're there for prestige or money or whatever. You shouldn't pursue psychiatry as a career, for any other reason than the fact that you genuinely care about people. Listening must be attached to *caring*. It's like a link. If you haven't got that real connection between listening and caring then we pick it up. And that's important to us, because it's usually from lack of caring that we've ended up in the situations we're in. That's what makes people with so-called 'mental illness' wary and untrusting of psychiatrists.

What feelings does it bring up for you when you are not listened to?

Frustration. Hopelessness. If psychiatrists don't listen and don't care then I'm not going to put my thoughts, ideas, feelings or energy into them; I don't want to say any more because it's just a waste of words.

It's also vital that the relationship with a therapist or psychiatrist is a two-way thing. You get psychiatrists who say, 'Oh I don't get attached to my clients; I won't allow myself to get attached.' My psychotherapist says that the way she sees it, it's almost impossible *not* to get attached and somewhat involved. She doesn't feel that you can have a good healing relationship with a client unless you take a certain amount of true interest and care. The respect must always go both ways.

I also think it is important that there is some level of commonality. This commonality can provide a basis for connection. For example, very early on in my relation-ship with my psychotherapist, we discovered that we both suffered from migraine headaches and took the same medication for them. That was a good foundation for beginning to understand each other.

What took you from the times of alienation and pain you described above, to that of the peace and contentment you have now?

I know it might sound bizarre but one of the first things to have an impact was a hug. A psychologist I was seeing hugged me and it really moved me. I had been raised in a family environment where people did not hug one another. I couldn't have cared less about receiving a hug or even whether anybody would want a hug from me. But when he hugged me, I experienced something that I simply had never had. I think I actually went through my series of appointments with that person to get the hug at the end!

What did the hug give you?

Warmth and a sense of belonging to the human race! I'd felt like a robot rather than a human being. It gave me a sense of 'Wow, I'm human and somebody in this world cares!' That hug was the closest anyone had ever come to me in my world and it made me feel an individual, a unique human being.

Do you feel you could have got that just from talking?

No. No. There's nothing that can touch the soul as much as physical contact. You can talk in great depth, but the touch of another human being is really special. I hadn't realised what a difference a genuine hug with genuine feeling behind it could make in your life. I hadn't realised how much you could begin to look at things differently . . . but apart from the hugs, he did give me the beginnings of *insight*, which, looking back on it, was at the very *root* of getting well. I began to understand that there were reasons for what was happening to me. Insight was the foundation of recovery.

But I must say, although the initial hug was great, it unsettled me. It made me very aware that there were feelings bubbling away underneath: feelings of anger. As much as I got out of the hug, there was a small part of me that began to feel that this person was getting a bit close. I was always afraid of getting too close to anyone, a professional person most of all. I was afraid they might want to enter my fantasy world and take it away from me. The thought of that made me paranoid because I didn't know what it would be replaced by.

Did you continue therapy with this psychologist?

No. I saw him for three years and I probably got as far as I could have at the time. Later I was referred to a public psychiatrist and she wanted me to see a private psychiatrist so that I could have some therapy. She referred me to my current psychiatrist who is also a practising psychotherapist. Her desire for me was that I didn't slip through the system. Those were her words to my psychotherapist: 'I don't want to see her slip through the system, because she's got far too much potential.'

The referring psychiatrist was later murdered, and I think we both saw it as a legacy that we had to fulfil. And I have no regrets. It was only a month or so before Christmas that my psychotherapist put her arms around me and said, 'You've come further than anyone else I've ever seen.' And that was one of those moments where my peace and contentment was touched by real happiness. They were words that I could never have dreamt would be said to me.

At the beginning it was very important to me that my psychotherapist was very similar to the person I had been searching for all my life. I was content to be with her because she was very close to me in age and personality. As I became more and more confident with her and as I learnt more coping skills, I began to give up little bits of the fantasy world and trust more of the real world.

As I see it now, it was important that I give it up. Some years after entering therapy, my psychotherapist confided in me that had I continued as I was, I would have ended up in a psychiatric hospital on a long-term basis. I'm very glad that I put in the work I did.

You spoke of learning coping skills. Was that an important part of your therapy?

Therapy was about everything, putting *everything* that had ever happened to me in my life into perspective. Good and bad. To understand it. To put it into a tense, whether that be present, past or future. To understand that some things happened then and aren't happening now, and that the *way* I'm feeling angry, upset or depressed about it *now* was because I didn't experience the feelings I should have at the time. I had bottled things up for 40 years and expressing them all those years later didn't lessen their intensity at all. It was just as traumatic as when it happened. But at the same time as all this I was also *trying* to see some sort of future for myself. It was a bit like unravelling a jumper into a big ball of wool and then trying to knit a new one out of it.

But I did begin to learn and develop life and coping skills: how to set boundaries for people, how to say 'no', how to ask for what I want, how to delegate things if I am burdened, how to ask for help . . . I never knew any of those things. I'll give you an example. I have a brother who is an alcoholic. From time to time he'd come to my home inebriated. He's a real handful when he's like that. Consequently I'd get extremely distressed and depressed. It never even occurred to me that I could set boundaries that he would have to abide by. I never thought I had the right. Because he was my brother I thought I had to put up with it.

But there came a point when I thought, 'Hang on, this is *my* house. This is *my* castle.' That was one of the most important and yet subtle understandings in the whole journey: to understand and appreciate my own home. *This* was mine. *This* was my sanctuary. My asylum. My place. My domain. Where I set the rules and I don't have to answer to anyone. A place of beautiful music, a garden, art mediums, crafts. And it was when I began to see all that, that I'd get a day here and there of peace and contentment. And I only had to experience one of those days to start believing that I could have that feeling for a week or a month! I was running towards a goal. I started to get excited.

Medication was also a part of therapy, but I would disagree with relying solely on medication. I am certain that we all have baggage and issues that interrupt our lives. Those issues can't possibly be solved by a tablet. You have to learn to deal with the issues themselves and put them away into some sort of order that is your own. It's ludicrous to think otherwise. But medication did alleviate some of the symptoms: the paranoia and depression. I still had admissions while taking medications but my admissions probably weren't quite as long because the symptoms weren't as severe.

It was important to me that my psychotherapist was *very* level-headed about medication. She insisted that at all times I knew what was best for me. She would encourage me to medicate myself and to judge for *myself* when I might need more medication or less. Similarly, if I was in hospital and I wanted to be released, the staff would ring her for an opinion. She would always say, 'If Joan says it's time to be released, then it's time to be released.' She insisted that I was the best judge in my own life and encouraged me to listen to myself. This was the opposite of my childhood.

Earlier on you used the word 'journey'.

Yes. It was like I was travelling in a spiral that was always moving onwards and upwards into infinity. I was always discovering new things about myself and about others. The view was forever changing. I never knew what I would see next, because I had never been there before.

But although in one way that journey was exciting and exhilarating, I also want to make the point that it is a very difficult journey. It can even be a *hell* of a journey. And it's not for the faint-hearted. In a sense, the less social life, outside activities and outer commitments, particularly during the difficult times, the better. You need to concentrate. You need to be alone and have a lot of private time to put into perspective what you've dealt with every week. I went weekly to therapy for ten years.

And along with psychotherapy, I also went to art therapy. I'd have my psychotherapy appointment late in the afternoon and then go to art the following morning, when everything was still fresh and full of feeling.

How did it come about that you pursued both art therapy and psychotherapy?

I'd been arty as a child, but I'd had to go out to work at fourteen and so I'd lost that in my life. But whenever I was admitted to hospital, the art room was the first place I would go. I've actually known my art therapist ever since my first admission.

The referring psychiatrist I had seen in the system had known I was creative. I had made some crafty gifts and things, and given them to her. She told my current psychotherapist that she thought it was important that I pursue this further. It is a known fact that it is important for people who suffer from so-called 'mental illness' to be arty and creative. With our sensitivities, it is very healing to tap into our creativity. I certainly know that I always feel much calmer and relaxed when I am being creative.

However, because I was seeing a psychiatrist privately,

I had to re-access the public system in order to gain access to the hospital's art therapy as an outpatient. I had to have a government social worker call on me. Another pre-requisite was that I could talk or write about what I had drawn. It was important that I was able to *interpret* my art. Once I had the concept of art therapy explained to me I never looked back. I would write pages upon pages.

How did the talking therapy and the art therapy work together?

There were no rules. There was no prescribed way that the therapy and the art went together. I'd talk about something in psychotherapy, I'd express whatever emotions were involved in the session, and then when I started to paint it I might realise that there was even more there than I could have known. At no point would I ever know what would come out.

Sometimes it was like the Mad Mouse: I got on, I didn't know where I was going, which way I was going to turn, what sort of feelings I would have. Every day was unique. Every day I valued. Every day I went to art was exciting.

Art also helped me to communicate. My communication skills had always been very poor, so until I could communicate better, the art was vital. I had always felt that I was like somebody with autism. I remember saying to both my psychotherapist and art therapist that I felt autistic. I *felt* it. I couldn't think of words. I couldn't get things out. I was shy. I was angry. It was all so complex.

The very first thing I ever drew was a mandala of my soul or inner self. In it there was turmoil. In my mandalas I use circles a lot. Any circles are about healing. Pyramids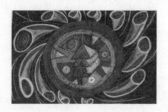

represent my spiritual side. After that first mandala, I made it a rule that from time to time I would do another one to see how I might have changed.

The very next week after the mandala, I did a drawing that was very constrained. It was like someone in a straight-jacket. It was the top of a ball shape divided by sections into lines and each section was coloured. I remember the art therapist asking, 'What does 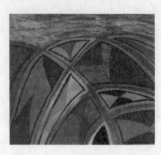 that represent to you?' It was easy to answer. It represented how I felt and how I saw the world. It was as though we were all confined to these box-like sections. Territorial. Not connecting. No room for eccentricities or difference. You have to fit here or here or here. If you fit anywhere else you are on the outer. It was like when I was a child. I didn't fit anywhere whereas all the other children in my family did.

Where has your particular use of symbols come from?

It's just something I feel for me.

. . . and the wide range of colours you use?

I probably use a lot of colour because I feel as if my whole life and all of who I am, is colourful. I have no problem using quite vibrant colours and plenty of them.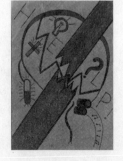

Did you also paint during times when you were feeling desperate or suicidal?

This drawing was done on a day I was feeling very suicidal. I wasn't sure how to bring everything together. It was as though I was stuck in a vicious circle – the medication (capsule), the spiritual side of my life (the cross), the brightness (the light globe), the confusion (the question mark), trying to move to the beat of my own drum (the drums) and the enemy (the snake). The red line through the middle was like my inner self snapping or breaking. I was feeling altogether very confused, very very angry and suicidal.

Could you show me other paintings that have a special significance for you?

I call this one *Time*. It looks very Indigenous because that's where I was at. I was going through psychotherapy, and struggling with who I was and what my beginnings were. As far as we know, 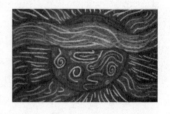 there could be some Indigenous blood in our family. My mother was born in the country in the 1920s, one of nine illegitimate children. My mother's father was listed as unknown but there was always talk of him being an Indigenous person. I've always felt a real connection with Indigenous people. I'm also a person who goes walkabout when I'm distressed. I'll lock up my house and walk. My mother did likewise.

Were you aware of its Indigenous quality when you were painting it?

No not initially. It was only something I was *feeling*. It was only pretty much when I saw the finished product that I looked at it and thought, 'Wow!'

What was the relevance of calling the work *Time*?

It was about going back in time in psychotherapy, but also the fact that time does heal.

This one is my favourite. I call it *The Collective Soul*. It's about thinking of people in a collective way. It's like a collection of happy souls of all shapes, sizes and colours that forms into a comet and trails off into infinity. Even 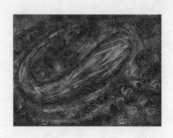 though some souls are hanging on to the tail, they are just as important as any other souls. Whether you're first, last or in-between, it just doesn't matter. Sometimes the collective soul loses some energy, but then it always re-generates, pulsating in size, colour and brightness. And that's what life is like.

I just love it. I *love* it . . . I was starting to feel good then. I thought, 'If I can feel this good, imagine how many other people could feel this if only given the opportunity'. To me, it's how it could be if more and more people are given the opportunities that I was. It can happen. And if it did happen . . . I wonder about how much happier, and brighter and more progressive the world would be . . .

Could you tell me more about the triptych at the opening of this interview?

The triptych makes me so happy because I remember the moment, the feeling, and the night I did it. It was at the time I had started to feel confident that the peace and contentment were really within my grasp. I was at home alone one night and I just felt . . . *peace!* And I went for the paper and the pastels and I just drew and drew and coloured and it came right out on the paper. It was as if I actually *felt and experienced* the whole sequence as it was happening . . .

The first drawing is the flower of the lotus or soul,

appearing or blooming. In the second, the flower opens even further to express rays of light and brightness and warmth. And in the third it goes on to release the white doves of peace. And as I drew those doves, it was almost like I felt them fly from within. It was as though I could feel their wings internally.

And then when I had finished, I lay them on the bed and I cried. I was really overwhelmed by it all. The feelings, the spontaneity, the colours . . . even the speed with which I had been able to get it down on paper amazed me. My hands must have been flying. It was one of the most beautiful things I have ever done.

As you were speaking of the doves I wondered if perhaps they were symbolic of that inner person you spoke of early in the interview.

Yeah. Yeah. As I was going through therapy, I was a bit like a snake that sheds skin after skin. Those skins were like the garbage and family clutter that I didn't need any more. And then after years and years, I finally got to a core . . . the heart of the matter. The soul. And this soul was freed by casting off all those skins. The doves were like that freedom flying out into the world. It was like being reborn.

We have something deep deep within us. Some connection with the universe. I now feel a wonderful connection with the very centre of the universe. It's almost like a pulse or a rhythm. It's like the rhythm of your life. The beat of your own drum.

I had my first full breakdown at the age of 27 and was admitted to hospital. I then went on to have countless admissions over the next years. It wasn't that things were happening, it was that I began to see that things were wrong. I began to realise how much I didn't know. One of the biggest shocks was that I realised I had no opinions of my own. I just hooked on to everyone else's opinions and ideas. 'I don't even have my own thoughts on how life began! Do I believe the Bible story or do I believe evolution?' I don't know how many admissions I had just trying to work that out. I knew I had to form some sort of opinion about that before I went anywhere. It was about working out the very basis of who I am. I thought that if I couldn't work that out, then I wouldn't get anywhere. I felt that if I didn't achieve some form of connection with things around me in my time here, then I would probably have to come back into this world again and live another life, and then another life . . . until I connected with the universe.

Did you form an opinion?

Yeah. And it was my own. And I felt good about it. And I've never altered it. It was that the journey of life is about self-development. You grow and you never stop. Within and without. As you grow within then it stands to reason that you'll grow outside of yourself as well.

Could you explain that a little more?

I'll give you an analogy. I read in an article an argument between theologists about whether God fills us up or whether we express God outwardly. And I think they're both right. The way I see it is that when your cup is full and running over, you can share it and give it away. Whatever or whoever God is . . . I see God as maybe a . . . gas. A gas or ether that fills you . . . then when you've got enough within and you feel complete (not euphoric or anything, just complete) then you can't but pass it on to others.

Does that imply that when you're still empty you can't connect with others?

Yeah. You won't connect. I didn't. I know that I didn't.

It's virtually impossible. For example, I've spent many Christmas Days on my own in my life because I always try to keep Christmas Day to spend with my brother. But because he may or may not get on the drink, I'm never really sure whether I'll spend it alone or with him. In years gone by, when I spent it alone, it didn't worry me. But the last two years, my world has expanded and I've moved more towards people. This year I had to spend Christmas alone and this year, for the first time, I felt lonely. *Really* lonely. I missed people.

What is it that people give you now?

Difference. It's the difference I enjoy. And that's the opposite of years ago. I didn't like that difference before; I wanted everyone to be the same as me. Same ideas. Same thoughts. Now I *love* to hear the difference of ideas, opinions and attitudes. I feel I've got the capability to appreciate people's difference. Even if I walk to the end of my street, I know that at least three people will stop, say hello and value my conversation. The ironic thing is that now I realise I wouldn't want anybody to be too much like me! It'd be pretty boring!

But as I've understood and appreciated the complexities, difference and uniqueness of other people, it's been really exciting to me that I've also connected better with my pets. In years gone by, they would have been 'just pets': animals that had to be fed and watered. I wouldn't have noticed their individual personalities and ways.

I also play a mentor role to young people. At the moment I have two young people in my life who look up to me. It has been something that has just happened. One has been diagnosed with a so-called 'mental illness'. I just offer them advice and conversation. I draw on all I have been through in my life. I feel that if I can help just one person, if I can change just one little corner or even half a street, then I will have served my purpose on the planet.

I feel so very sad that governments only look at people with so-called 'mental illness' in an economic way, because if only more people had access to the sort of help that I've had, so many more people could be saved. I see so many people who are quite literally 'lost souls'. And it's heartbreaking. If you talk to them, you know without a doubt that each and every one has just as much potential as I ever did.

I feel so very grateful to all the people who have helped me along the way and I think it's important to say that it's not only *me* who they've helped and healed. It has flowed on. It is like a stone that has been thrown into a pond. The ripples go out and out.

If circumstances had been different, I may have suicided or I may have ended my days in a psychiatric hospital . . . but now I consider myself a valuable member of the community.

If you had one thing you could say to your 27-year-old self, from the perspective of your 56-year-old self, what would it be?

Don't take it all too seriously. No matter what confronts you, it's not the end of the world. There seems to be a natural course of events in life that strips away the earthly things and the seriousness we place on them. If we could just look within ourselves and learn to connect more with the very inner spirit or soul, then we would cling less to every little thing that goes wrong.

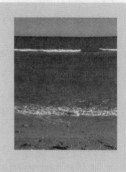

Dimitri

Dimitri is 28 years old. He is an honours university student and his interests include philosophy and spirituality, social frameworks and politics, art and culture. He plays guitar and writes poetry.
'I like the ocean – life is like an ocean of experience.'

I don't know if I've ever suffered a mental illness as such but . . .

I had a fairly long-term relationship that ended. I had also been working in a very busy government bureaucracy and it was pretty stressful. I had realised that the office world wasn't for me and that I was just doing it for the money. It was starting to really eat at me. I'd always been creative in terms of music and writing. I had done a film degree but then I'd ended up in an occupation where I really couldn't express myself. I felt I wasn't fulfilling my potential. I knew something had to change and I wasn't sure how that was going to happen.

About a year after the relationship ended, I started planning to return to university to do my honours in film. At that time I'd also started to ask myself for assistance to get help with my life.

What do you mean by assistance?

Just sort of personally. I wrote some letters to my inner self. I'd try to tap into myself to open up different paths in my life.

One day, after I'd arranged to take leave from work, I was at a friend's house and I had an intuition that I could go home and just tune in. I went home and lay on my bed. I'd previously had out-of-body experiences and I thought that this was something like that. I projected inwards, into myself, rather than outwards and I just had a very full-on experience.

Images started coming up. A very strong image of a tree arose and it felt as though it was my very Being. I had a sense that there was an intense pyramid shape that was drawing me towards it, and as it did so, it was as though part of me had to die and another part had to remain here. With that I also had intense images of people that I knew. I felt the connections between us. I was saying to myself that I *did* want to stay in this world with these people and that I didn't want to die completely. I wanted to stay and fulfil this life. As the experience continued there was an image of a wavering circular pattern in space that I felt came into my Being and I had the sense that it was like a new identity. Then I experienced a kind of hot intense point or dot in space that was humming with a certain sort of sound. It started to zoom or focus me in and then it opened out into the life of a guy in America. I assumed that this was another life I was living, like a counterpart or alternate self or something. I felt that I was directly contacting a different part of myself. Towards the end of the experience I felt that I was heading into the sun – it was like a light of consciousness or pure awareness. For a while it was as though I literally had the sun within my head. It felt like I had touched the Source. It was so intense that I could understand how countless worlds and beings could erupt from it.

The images continued for about an hour.

When I came out of it I was pretty rattled. Although in some way the experience had been exhilarating and exciting, and I felt I had contacted a deeper or larger part of myself, my everyday ego felt off-centre. I didn't really understand what had happened. Although I knew I had touched something, I also feared that I may have gone terribly mad, because I couldn't really assimilate the experience into a normal context. I was also terrified because the intensity was beyond anything I had ever experienced or even heard of. It's not easy to relate because I don't think there's a way to describe that sort of experience in words. It was like walking into a foreign country and thinking, 'Wow this is pretty incredible but I can't really make much sense of it.'

Were you able to return to your everyday life?

I went to work the next day and I felt different. The work environment started to look surreal – as though it was a camouflage system. The experience was so strong that it blurred my perception of everyday reality. Perhaps it was a bit like an acid trip, but I've never been into that sort of stuff. Then, when I was looking into the computer, I started to feel dead. I told my co-ordinator that I felt really out of it and that I had to go home. I couldn't drive because I was having a panic attack of sorts, so someone drove me home. My normal sense of who I was had been really jolted.

What *was* your normal sense of who you were?

That I was just the normal working person, an office worker, but also with a striving to explore things a bit more deeply. From the time I was a teenager I'd done a lot of reading into spirituality and philosophy. Perhaps it was lucky that I had that basis. Perhaps in part it was this reading that had led me to this experience, because it was a direct experience and expression of a lot of the stuff that, up until that point, I had only understood intellectually. I had read about concepts like alternate realities, multi-dimensional personhood and the nature of consciousness and now I was experiencing them. I was brought into an inner space that was way beyond my ordinary self. It gave me a sense that there was much more to who I am. It changed how I saw myself.

What happened when you got home from work that day?

Well I took a couple of days off. I thought I'd really flipped out. I didn't know what to call it.

Eventually, the human resources co-ordinator at work realised that I'd had a bit of a breakdown and suggested that I go and see a counsellor. Not being into conventional psychology and having taken my own road, I wasn't really keen on the idea, but because I was so rattled I thought I might give it a try. So I went to a counsellor at a privately contracted place. From the moment I got in there I didn't feel comfortable. I didn't feel she would be able to relate to my experience.

Did you tell her about the experience?

I went through it a bit. I said I'd had a breakdown, was stressed out at work and had a relationship break-up earlier in the year. I also told her that I'd done a lot of reading and done a bit of philosophy.

She started asking me about my parents' separation and I just started to lose the thread. I really wasn't into the idea. I had dealt with my parents' separation in my own way years ago. I was aware of my feelings around it. My parents were married for 25 years and they used to separate quite regularly. Once every year or two they separated for a while. I was used to it. I was aware of the impact.

What did the counsellor say?

Well she told me about this therapy . . . some light-

flashing therapy . . . some sort of neuronal therapy . . .
I just thought, 'This doesn't feel right to me.'

What was this therapy meant to do?

I don't really know. Help me get over things I guess.
All I knew was that it didn't feel right and that the context
in which she was trying to place my experience was
wrong. She gave me some pamphlets about this therapy
and I just left there and the first thing that popped into
my head was the idea of going to see an old counsellor
who I'd seen when I was younger. My parents had had
family sessions with him and I had gone along to a couple
of those. Once or twice I had also gone to him with
my own personal issues – about being a teenager and
trying to work things out. I'd felt a connection with him
from when I was younger.

You went to see him?

Yes. He basically listened to me a lot and affirmed
my experience. The sense he gave me was that although
I'd had a pretty full-on experience, it was going to
reconnect me in a way. I had always been very caught
up in my head, and during the experience I had an
impulse to try and connect with my body more . . . to
send this energy down from my head and into the rest
of my body. I told him about that and he said, 'Exactly.
That's what you need to do. You need to connect with
your body.' Rather than a breakdown, he suggested it
had been a break*through*.

He also had an understanding of the sorts of philosophy and spirituality that I'd been reading. He gave me a
framework within which to understand the experience
that was a bit deeper than conventional frameworks. He
also said that I had the framework to understand it within
myself. He said that some people who may be termed
schizophrenic might have similar experiences but they

wouldn't have the framework within which to understand them or be able to come out of them and maintain an everyday sense of self. I felt I'd been dealing with questions ever since I was younger that were a bit deeper than your everyday experiences of 'getting on with life'.

Questions about the meaning of life?

That's right. What we are and what I was. I guess everyone asks them at some stage in their life – perhaps during a mid-life crisis or after a relationship breakdown. I'm sure it's interrelated, as to why these experiences emerge. I think it's difficult for a lot of us to combine physical and spiritual reality, and I felt that through this process I might be bringing those together. I don't think I was always operating from a true sense of who I felt myself to be. Like a lot of us, I had a lot of idealised self-conceptions: what I *should* be like, what I *should* be doing, how things *should* have gone or what I *should* be understanding at a certain time. Those were obviously starting to break down in a big way.

Interestingly, after I had this experience I refused to take any kind of medication – I didn't believe that there was anything truly wrong with me. I couldn't deny the experience. I felt it was meaningful. Although it had freaked me out I had a faith that there would be a positive outcome in the long run.

Did you eventually go back to work?

I went back to work to tidy up some bits and pieces and arranged to take my leave early. I said I'd had a breakdown or a meltdown. I was pretty shaky for a month or two and after that I slowly entered a state of depression where I started to sink into things. That's when I actually started to feel a bit better and that's when I went back to university; even though I didn't feel particularly solid, I wanted to give it a try.

How did it go at university?

It was fairly hard. It was difficult interacting with people, and I'd never had that difficulty before. I was normally very sociable and formed close relationships, but this was different. I had come back after being away for a long time and didn't know the people there, but it was also because I'd had this experience and gone into depression.

What was it about your interaction with people that had changed?

My sense of self was no longer solidified. It was all over the place and I was generally anxious. It made it hard to even have the desire to contact people or get to know people intimately. I felt like I needed a lot of time out for myself . . . to sit on the lounge and do a bit of reading or take in what I'd gone through and to try to work out why it had happened.

What do you think might have happened had you not had a framework within which to put this experience?

If I hadn't found someone who I could connect with and who had an understanding of what I had been through, I am really not sure that I would have got through it. I don't know how you can fit that sort of experience into an everyday framework, even an everyday psychological framework. I had some knowledge of various kinds of outlooks, self-help books and psychologies. I had grown up in that sort of environment to some extent and I think that this was a vital key to normalising my experience.

My parents were really supportive, and it was probably also important that I had close friends who had had similar kinds of experiences. I think it's critical to have *someone* who has an understanding, like a guide who affirms your experience. When you look at psychology, the standard approach is that there is something wrong with you and they're going to fix you up. That's not ever how I felt. The concept of being broken or having something wrong with my brain just didn't apply. I thought there was great personal meaning in it for me.

What has happened since then?

The actual breakdown was only about a year and half ago. I started to see my counsellor fairly regularly, every couple of weeks, or whenever I felt I needed it. I had also gone into quite an intense depression. I felt like taking time out. I wasn't sure of a lot of things – what I wanted to do with my life and who I was. I knew I had had this experience and I knew I wasn't going to be able to understand it overnight. I also started to realise that I hadn't wanted to be at work for a long time. I realised that I'd probably been depressed for quite some time and had been fighting it. My counsellor gave me some specific articles about depression that were totally and utterly life saving.

What did they say?

The basic approach of the articles was that depression was something that was actually beneficial if you could accept it and go through it, even if it wasn't necessarily comfortable; that depression was a deepening process during which a lot of the questions and notions you had about yourself and about life needed to be taken in deeply and felt, rather than just thought about and questioned.

I think there needs to be a broader understanding that depression is natural. Considering the wars that are happening, the social contexts that people live in and the world situation, it would almost be crazy if people weren't depressed. In the West I think we live in a very surface culture and we have a sort of 'meaning void'. I think depression is perhaps a natural way to find that meaning. I don't think the standard nine-to-five lifestyle and the 'buying happiness' thing is fulfilling for people. Other people had breakdowns at work, and maybe that's telling us something about the social fabric we live in. Perhaps we need to find out more about the nature of what it is to be human and what meaning is for people.

Those articles gave you a personal understanding that what you were going through was meaningful. How did that affect your approach to feeling depressed?

I didn't feel that I had to fight it. I didn't feel that I shouldn't be feeling the way that I was. I didn't feel that I needed to go and get some sort of fixing. I spent a lot of time just lying down on the couch, tuning into myself and letting things just come to me. I began to understand that depression is a part of life and that you can't always be 'up-and-at-'em'.

So that was all very much the opposite of the 'shoulds' that you mentioned earlier.

Very much so. When I reflect now I think it was a big part of the reason I had that sort of breakdown. Or breakthrough. It actually enabled me to a large extent, though not completely, to just let go of that and let myself work things out naturally without *trying* so vigilantly to work them out in my head all the time.

Are you still going to uni?

Well going to uni was pretty difficult. I saw my doctor and explained where I was at, so that I could get some medical certificates to go down to part-time study. That was quite trying. I almost completely withdrew, but my co-ordinator at uni was quite supportive and gave me the extra time I needed. I hung in there and thought, 'I'm going to make this film. I'm going to give it a go.'

And I started to get into the film and then I met my new girlfriend and I was really happy about that.

What is your film about?

Basically that you recontact yourself through depression. I guess it's a bit autobiographical. The main character has a lot of issues and concerns in life, goes into depression, has a breakdown and is transformed through that. He ends up being different and happier, so to speak.

Life informing art . . .

Yes. I hope to be able to use my experiences creatively . . . but I've been struggling to finish off the script. And I'm still at that stage now. It's been very up and down. Trying to balance a relationship, to know how I feel in terms of my relationship and also in terms of the film work is difficult. I'm questioning a lot of things like love and connection . . . I've questioned all my relationships throughout my life. But it's not just questions, it's direct feelings . . . like how I *feel* things is different now.

Does that difference bring with it the positive outcome that you had intuited might come through this experience?

I do feel different a lot of the time and I do appreciate that difference and feel a lot stronger and more myself, but there are times when I also feel shakier as well and worry that I may be losing it more.

I feel fundamentally that I've been going through a kind of birth. Other aspects of myself that I haven't been able to experience in my life are coming through. I guess like a birth it's quite painful as well. And unsettling and scattered. I feel all over the place in a lot of ways. It's like having a lot of various moods, and sometimes I feel okay and other times I feel like I just can't deal with things or I don't understand. I hope I'll eventually come through that process so that I get to a more stable ground and feel like I'm acting from a more authentic self.

Could you explain a little more what you mean by 'acting from a more authentic self'?

Acting from my authentic feelings and being able to express how I feel towards certain people in certain relationships. Before I hadn't really questioned or thought about it that much. Right in the middle of it now, I can't say that it is particularly pleasant all the time because I don't feel solidified; I'm still learning just to trust that authentic flow. In modern social contexts it's very hard for people to trust that authentic flow and I think that's one of the big reasons why so many people have breakdowns and experience depression. Those greater life questions that people ask aren't really faced directly.

I have to face it that it may not be easy for quite a while, in terms of relationships, connecting and going about my everyday life. I could really sum up the experience by saying that although it's been up and down, it's also been very transformative.

Cheryl

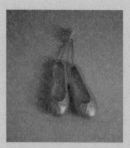

Cheryl is 40 years old. Flowers. Roses. English rose gardens. Lots of colour . . . *'The photo is of pink ceramic ballet shoes that hang on my wall. They represent me at probably age five, when we'd just moved from Wales to Liverpool. It was a reasonably good time in my life. My mother decided to enrol me in ballet classes and from that moment I had a love of dance and movement. I had little pink ballet shoes, little pink soft slippers . . . I never forgot those. I became a dancer later in my teens. I went to dance and drama college for three years. And again that was a good time in my life.*

Later I lost my love of all things pink and 'ballet' . . . I forgot about those little things that meant something to me. When the pink came back I felt a direct connection back to those good times. I now recall those times when I am feeling low.'

Repression

The place for me to start is when I was eleven years old. I remember the date because it was my birthday. I had the sudden realisation that my life wasn't quite right. It happened for only a split second, but that one thing has sustained me to this point. It was a little bit of humanity that enabled me to stay alive as long as I have.

Whenever I got to a point at which I thought, 'Okay, this is it, I'm going to die today,' that realisation pulled me back. It gave me a vision of something else . . . that there *was* something else. I didn't know what that something else was, but I knew that the way it was all happening wasn't how it was meant to be: we weren't allowed to go out on the street, we weren't allowed to have friends in the house, we had the curtains drawn, the phone wouldn't be answered, we checked who was at the door before opening it . . . that wasn't right . . . how would I know that as an eleven-year-old girl? It was a feeling inside of me. If I hadn't had that, I would have accepted everything and been swallowed up by it. I would not have had anything to measure my life against.

But although that was a defining moment for me, there were also other moments. When I was in my early twenties I was very promiscuous. I had no idea why I was sleeping with every person I met and why I had no boundaries at all, sexual or otherwise. At that point I had a similar feeling inside: 'You're going to have to do something about this.' But I thought that maybe I'd do it later. Again it happened for only a moment and then it was gone . . . and I carried on. I had no idea what it was all about: drinking, taking drugs, the whole sex thing and having no thought of personal safety. The number of situations I put myself in that were dangerous and that I could have died! But I had no idea.

I now look back and see that they were coping strategies, survival techniques. In England I had been an actress, on the stage and on TV, and even *that* was my survival technique for about ten or fifteen years. I could go out on stage and become someone else. It was fabulous. I never had to be myself. There was always a façade around me. The only time I fell apart was between rehearsals or after performances when I had to be in the world.

I met an actress from Jamaica and we became very close friends. I realised that there was something completely disjointed, jangly and unpredictable about her. I was drawn to it but at the same time it also repelled me. One night she suddenly told me that at age five she had been raped by an uncle in Jamaica. The minute she said it, I had an overwhelming feeling that I had to get away from her. I completely divorced myself from her.

I forgot about it for a long time. When I was in hospital after giving birth to my first son in 1990, there was a woman in the next cubicle who told me her partner had been abusing her daughter from another relationship. Again . . . I cut that relationship off.

But when my daughter was born in 1999 it was like, 'I've got a *girl*'. I was looking at a smaller version of myself and suddenly it felt like a freight train had hit me. I remember waking up my husband one night and saying, 'Oh my god, I've been repressing something.' I was absolutely terrified. It was like little bits had been coming out over the years, but in having a daughter I knew that I wouldn't be comfortable having any males around her. I had become aware that my reaction to men was to switch off and try to escape. For a long long time if I met a man of African descent on a train or on a bus I would have *the* worst panic attacks. I couldn't breathe. I thought he was going to rape or kill me and had no idea what it was about.

The birth of my daughter was the moment my real life started, because I was suddenly hit with the reality of who I was. Until that moment my life had been a sham, it was nothing . . . At the time though, it felt like the beginning of the end because I had no conscious understanding of who this new person was. It was like it was happening to a third person . . . somebody over there. It felt like I was less than I was before. I had always felt that I wasn't worth much, but now I felt like I was worth even less. At least before I had an identity: I was someone's wife, I was an actress, I was somebody's mother.

It wasn't till the birth of my younger son two-and-a-half years later that everything just crumbled. His birth had been particularly difficult and we almost lost him. Afterwards I just kept getting more and more depressed. The doctor told me it was because of the difficulties surrounding his birth, but then one day I just snapped. I was hysterical. I grabbed the cord of the breast pump machine and tied it around the light fitting and tried to hang myself. My husband called the ambulance and I went to hospital, and they assumed antidepressants would fix it. Then I tried to hang myself again. I was driven by it. When you want to die you want to die. They drugged me up to the eyeballs and put me in the lock-up for a week.

Were there any words with that 'wanting to die'?

It was a feeling . . . 'I can't live'. With his birth had come more memories and the worst devastation of remembering who and where and when . . . My father was the main person I remembered . . . and a couple of his brothers who came to our house . . . I couldn't envisage a life beyond that remembering . . . The first thing that came to me were my uncle's eyes; I didn't like the look in them. But my father kept insisting that I go and sit on his lap . . . and that was where the cutting off of my wants and needs started . . . because my father was also a very violent man and we were regularly beaten for very minor infractions. Along with what happened in an inappropriate sexual manner, there was also that violence and the threat of it. The punishment wasn't just about keeping the child out of danger, it was the intent . . . it wasn't about teaching me, it was about venting whatever it was within him.

He would always say, 'This is for your own good.' He would say, 'You're not listening to me, so this is what's going to happen.' He had these great big pieces of post with which he would chase us around the house, and if you ran it would be worse for you. I could never stand still because it would be like waiting for the executioner, so he would have to come and drag me from under the bed and beat me with a stick.

Did he treat everyone in the family in this way?

I remember my two older brothers were hit and beaten, but it was mainly reserved for the girls. My sister was diagnosed with autism and also had an eating disorder. She wouldn't eat and my father would beat her to try to make her eat. At one stage she had started talking just a little bit, but after one particularly bad beating she never spoke again. He also beat my mother on a regular basis. I remember one occasion he blackened her eye and threw her clothes in the fire. The police were called. My mother took us to live with our grandmother for a while after that. She eventually went back to him, but over the years the violence continued.

Could you tell me more about the general environment in which you grew up?

My parents were of mixed race. My father was of African descent and my mother was from Ireland and they migrated to Liverpool, where we were brought up. We had an enormous mix. My mother's parents were Catholic and Protestant and fought constantly and then there was the added fact that my father was black in 1960s Liverpool.

There were six of us children, although my mother had eight pregnancies. One child was stillborn and the other was a late miscarriage. Looking back I think those losses affected her dreadfully. She also suffered from severe postnatal depression after the birth of my youngest brother. I remember after one birth she had needed a blood transfusion and was convinced that someone's spirit had entered her body.

But the main thing was the disharmony. All the time. There was always *something*. We never had a day that there wasn't any shouting or drama. The days that we didn't have drama were the days we went to the zoo or the safari park. We knew that when we were away from the house we had to look like the picture of the perfect family.

Meanings

When I was working I couldn't deal with the interactions. When there are a lot of people in a situation I am very good at finding out who I have to please, but it is at the expense of who I am. I *become* my feelings. There is no 'I'. If I was upset at work, I just became 'upset'. If I became angry, I just became that anger. The interactions became too much.

I had a very different identity at work. I was a woman who was still married, still living at home with my children . . . but that had begun to unravel. There was one woman at work who was a filmmaker. I felt quite close to her and we had a lot in common. Towards the end I was beginning to cut back my hours and there were times I was really 'talky' and over-the-top. I felt that I had to qualify my behaviour and so I told her I was 'mentally ill'. I told her that I was really comfortable telling her this, but I actually wasn't. She stopped calling and another person at work soon found out too. I was devastated and felt violated.

Then someone at work accused me of doing something I hadn't done. That tied in with all my childhood stuff – of being punished for things I didn't do.

I was in the car park and I had called the crisis service and told them that I knew I needed help, that I couldn't see and that I was going to drive my car over the edge. And so they sent the police in. And then people at work saw the police escorting me to hospital and I was so humiliated. Up until that time my husband had been my support system, but he had broken his ankle two days earlier, so he was out of action. That completely threw me. I couldn't cope with him being out of action. I was taken into a cubicle and was left there. Eventually I started to feel very unsafe and panicky so I just got up and left, went home, tied a cord around my neck and was fully hoping not to wake up in the morning.

Then I heard a banging on my door and it was the police. They took me back to hospital. The nurses were extremely angry that I'd left. They wanted to give me an injection. I said that I didn't want an injection but rather wanted someone to listen to me. They told me I was hysterical and so I became those feelings. I *became* hysterical. A security guard grabbed me and they strapped me to a bed. They gave me the injection and I was left there for the night. Then at one stage I just wanted to turn over and go to sleep and so I slipped my arm out of one of the restraints. The guard saw me and thought I was trying to get out. I said, 'Look I'm calmer now . . .' and I became conscious of playing their game. I said, 'Look I'm really sorry, but I just want to go to sleep now.' I knew I had to play the game to get what I needed. I was detained for 48 hours because I had escaped.

That night I tried to strangle myself with the hose from an oxygen bottle. A nurse even saw that my face was bright red, but she merely assumed that I must have been out in the sun too long! But when the professor came in the following day I made sure I was as calm as anything. In my mind I was all over the place but I knew I just wanted to get out of there. I made a decision right there and then that this was never going to happen to me again. When you go looking for help you don't expect to be railroaded into decisions that are better for *them*. Nobody was listening to me and anybody with half a brain could see that I was absolutely traumatised. At one stage they started to bring up all my history of abuse and they just expected me to be unaffected by it.

They saw no meaning in your behaviour . . .

None. I felt it was *all* meaningful. I felt that there was a reason for it *all*. Something was driving me. I had an overwhelming sense of being driven by *something*. But I didn't know yet what that meaning or reason was. If you don't *know* yourself and if you don't know what you are feeling, these behaviours seem to come from nowhere. All you know is that your body is no longer able to suppress everything and it comes out however it will.

You're like a jigsaw puzzle that hasn't been finished. There are pieces lying everywhere and it is as though they're asking you to put it together with pieces from another puzzle. You're trying to piece together what your life means but you have two separate lots of pieces from which to make one puzzle.

In that hospital environment, trained people were no real help. They had *no* idea . . . they weren't engaging me . . . they weren't looking for it . . . they weren't even allowing me to engage *them*. . . . I knew it was all wrong but what do you do? In the end you are basically informed about your behaviour by the reaction of people around you. They tell you whether it is good or bad, when it actually isn't either. It's just their opinion.

Do you feel the only interest of the hospital staff was to control your immediate behaviour?

Yes. That's right. And I saw that in many other

instances. When I was in the lockup after the birth of my son, a girl called Laura was there. A nurse had told me that she had been taking drugs and was a bit psychotic. I'd never heard the word 'psychotic' before and assumed it meant that she was a bit stoned. I remember she was staring at me through a sort of unbreakable glass window, and I couldn't tolerate it, so I went up to the glass and screamed at her, 'What do you want?' They ended up restraining Laura. Later the nurse explained to me that she was a bit intrusive because of what was going on for her, but that in a few days she would calm down and be quite different.

Sure enough a couple of days later we talked and she told me about her relationship with her mother: her mother didn't want anything to do with her. I told her about my situation and we ended up bonding. Towards the end of her time there Laura had phoned her mother from the unit, and her mother had said, 'Why are you calling me? I don't want to hear from you.' She came to me and told me how devastated she was.

Later when we were watching TV Laura started getting wound up and talking really loudly and the staff told her to keep quiet. However, the situation escalated and she ended up breaking the glass window with a chair. The staff dragged her, restrained her, medicated her and sent her off to B . . ., an horrendous place at the psychiatric hospital. I was so incensed. The staff knew about the phone call with her mother but they didn't have the common sense to ask if she wanted to talk about it. They saw her behaviour as disruptive and that was as far as it went. They saw no connection between the two incidents. There was no thinking about it. I tried to talk to the nurse about it the next day, but she just gave me stock answers. She didn't respond to me like a human being, she responded to me like I'd pressed a button and asked a robot what the correct answer was.

Had you seen yourself as 'mentally ill' before that episode at work?

It went in waves. When things got really tough I thought there must be something wrong with me and I must be really sick. My emotions would spiral out of control and that would continue on for days. I would get completely overwhelmed. I couldn't cope with a simple interaction or if the car broke down, so I thought I must be 'mentally ill'. My first suicide attempt was at fifteen and whenever things spiralled out of control I took an overdose. I thought that's what you did when you got really upset about something . . . you tried to kill yourself. I probably had ten or fifteen attempts. Other moments when I was calm and rational, I thought I was just feeling my emotions and that there was nothing wrong that.

Had you ever been given a diagnosis?

My suicide attempts up until then had always been in an environment that protected me from professionals: with friends, after a one-night stand . . .

And now?

When my second son was six weeks old, I was taken off to a place for new mothers. My behaviour was called 'disruptive' because I was 'upsetting the other mothers'. I tried to tell them about what was happening with me but they didn't want to hear it. Everything kept going back to my childhood particularly my inability to tolerate any form of authority. They threatened to lock me in a ward and keep my baby away from me and at that time the doctor casually threw 'borderline personality disorder' at me. That actually provided more questions than answers for me; there was no medication and no information.

A few weeks later, after another suicide attempt I was in the hospital's psychiatric ward and I was given another diagnosis, bipolar affective disorder and I was given mood stabilisers. For a few weeks I was a bit trippy but okay, so they released me. Then for about five or six months I was on a huge dose of a mood stabiliser and I didn't realise that I was completely zonked out. I had no recollection of what it was like to laugh or have a basic level of energy to carry on normally. I was sleeping the whole time. They had me where they wanted me. They booked me in with a worker and the first thing he said to me was that I shouldn't get attached to him because I could only see him for a limited number of weeks. I thought, 'Whoa . . . I've just come here and you don't even know anything about me . . . and you're already laying out the rules of what I have to do to get what I need!' Whenever I went to these places it was as though they were trying to fit me in with their diagnoses; fit me in with who they wanted me to be. It was never about me as a human being.

What do you mean when you use the words 'human being'?

That I'm not just my body. I'm not just my behaviour. I'm not just what I say. I'm complex. There's a lot to me. There's emotions involved. There's where I have come from . . . And 'why' is important . . . the *meaning* of it. For instance, I've got diabetes; but it's not because I'm overweight. That may have *caused* it, but it's not why!

What do you see as the 'why' in terms of your diabetes?

It's a learning tool for me. It's a healing thing for me. It's saying: 'This is your body, and you need to love

145

you, you need to accept you, and only when you do that will you be well.'

Do you also see 'mental illness' as a learning tool?

Oh god yeah . . . I've learnt more about me and about the world through this than anything . . . the humanity through just being with other human beings and hopefully contributing to their lives. Like with Laura . . . there was a camaraderie there. It's about meeting other people in my situation. It's like we're the aliens and we've got a secret code and a secret language and *they're* the earthlings and they don't understand what we're talking about.

I just found more truth, more connectedness . . . each time I've had a hospitalisation there's been a person, or there's been a moment that's informed me just that little bit more about *me*. There's no bullshit. People tell you things about their lives that *mean* something. But I also learnt about getting around the system, not in a devious way, but in a way that was productive for me. Rather than the psychiatrists or the medications it was my interactions with other patients that informed my behaviour and helped me.

Staying alive

When I was in hospital I discovered a song by Michael Franti called *Stay Human*. The words from that song reflected the place I was in. I played them over and over. When I listened to that song, I realised I was not alone and nor was I strange or weird. What I was going through wasn't just *my* struggle . . . it was a *universal* struggle. That thought kept me alive.

Living alone

Last August I had my tonsils removed, and the hospital gave me large doses of painkillers. A couple of days later I was at home and my husband said, 'You look very grey.' I remember saying, 'Help me.' I thought I said it really loudly, but afterwards he told me it was barely audible. The ambulance was called. I was unconscious and they tried to revive me. I was in intensive care for three days and almost lost my life. At one stage my husband decided to go and play cricket and I realised I was alone. I thought, 'If I die now, there's nobody here. It's just me.'

I realised that it *was* just me. It doesn't matter how many people I have in my life to support me and love me, it was just *me*. If I can't do things in my life for myself then it doesn't matter. I realised that I couldn't go back to living at home with him and being in a co-dependent relationship. I decided to live on my own.

It was important for me to separate from my husband and children to find out who I was and find out what I wanted from my life. Being away from them is huge for me. I have since discovered that I was putting a lot of my identity into them. They were filling a need in me and as long as I needed them in that way, I couldn't have the relationship with them I wanted. It's no wonder that I think life is not worth living because I don't have a foundation; I don't have a substance to my life. I can't be a mother at the moment, I can't raise my children, because I have nothing there. It feels like I am a baby again. In fact I think my behaviour has become very baby-like: I have long sleeps, I allow myself to sit at the computer all night . . .

I think it's part of not putting restrictions on myself, because whenever I want to do something like that there's always a voice saying: 'No, you've got to do this or that.' I want to be a child again. I want to be able to say, 'No, I don't want to eat my dinner' or 'I want to have ten million lollies.'

Starting again?

Yes, very much starting again. I think it's no accident that I am living alone without the distractions of work or family. I am learning to be with *me*. Throughout my whole life there has been noise: other people's noise, other people's influence on me, other people's ideas about me . . . that I'm too fat, that I'm too this or too that. Being in relationships I always focused on the other person and put myself aside. I never ever had *me*. Coming away from the noise I had to learn to sit with a silence that was just mine. If noise or other people's voices came into my head I could work out what was theirs and what was mine.

What was the silence like initially?

Terrifying. I was more suicidal in those first few months than ever before. I couldn't bear it. For the first few months the noises were louder than when I had been with people. I didn't know what to do. There was constant chattering with every single thing I did. I was always contradicting myself, criticising myself . . .

When I didn't have the constant chatter I spent days lying on the floor wondering, 'How am I ever going to get up tomorrow?' I didn't see the point. I was about to turn 40 and I had nothing to show. My whole life had been a train wreck. I didn't understand the decisions I'd made, I didn't *like* the decisions I'd made and yet they were with me.

They didn't feel like decisions *you* had made?

They were based on nothing I can think of as coherent or as tangible and yet I had to take responsibility for them. I felt a great deal of anger about that. How do you take responsibility for something that had no foundation? 'Oh I think I'll just have a child!' 'Oh I think I'll just travel overseas!' They came from nowhere. I simply followed whatever popped into my head; there was no deeper sense of *me* behind them.

Did the chattering die down?

It didn't fully stop. When it did start to quieten down, I was so used to the adrenalin and the drama that I immediately looked for distractions. I thought, 'Oh my god, if there's nothing to worry about, then why be here?' I started focusing on my husband, telling myself that I really wanted to be with him . . . although I didn't. I decided I needed the money for a car so that I could visit the children, so I got a job at a call centre and fitted back into my work identity.

For the first month or so work distracted me, but I *knew* there was a difference within me. I was back where I was, but with a different awareness. I could no longer just *react* to life and to situations . . . I couldn't do that any more. I had information, I had knowledge about myself . . . I *knew* it wasn't for me. I did not want to be there. I was aware that my body was just going through the motions . . . I had three hospitalisations while I was there.

And what happened when you left?

Huge realisation and huge relief . . . I suddenly stopped. I could no longer continue taking on every environment around me . . .

What sort of relationship do you have with silence now?

I have a pretty good relationship with silence. I realise that I filled the silence with talk and chatter because I felt uncomfortable. When I am with my eldest son I can now allow the silence to just be there and it gives him permission to fill that space. He naturally wants to talk now. If my intention is to talk to him because I am uncomfortable he will pick up on that and he won't talk back. If I am just comfortable with the silence he will sense that it is okay for him to talk. The silence is giving me a space and everyone around me a space.

The silence is something satisfying now. It is like that moment of satisfaction when you are very thirsty and you take that first drink. It is the stillness on the water on a warm day. The stillness is still a scary place, but in it I am beginning to find clarity. I can make decisions that are *my* decisions. The silence gives me the space to listen to myself.

Healing

The first psychiatrist I was sent to, told me I was 'too difficult' for her. I had just finished telling her about my horrendous childhood and she said, 'Oh, I'll stop you there . . . I won't be able to help you.' It was surreal. It was like a cartoon.

When I came out of there I was a complete mess. I was crying. There was this sense of, 'If I get anywhere *near* what you are offering here then I can't cope with you'. And that went back to that abandonment as a child . . . that abandonment by my parents: 'You're too much. Be quiet. Don't sing. Children should be seen and not heard.'

But all the same, I didn't agree with her; I didn't agree that I *was* 'too difficult'. I felt it was outrageous. She had an opportunity to assist a person and she denied it. I wondered why she was in that job . . . this woman sitting in her office with a white leather lounge suite that she was terrified of me sitting on! I could see her looking me up and down . . .

But I also remember thinking, 'If this is too difficult for you then maybe my healing does not lie outside of me. Perhaps there is something *inside* me that is going to be better medicine than anything out there.' I am the expert on me. Whatever there is of me, I know it better than anybody out there. I am living it. That was healing for me because it was important to make that distinction.

Do you know what sort of people she *did* work with?

Obviously money was a driving force for her. When I first went in there I had asked if she bulkbilled because I was in receipt of a pension. She said, 'Well for some people I do . . .' and as soon as she said that I knew that she was going to make a decision about who she wanted to see and who she didn't.

I recognise discrimination because I have had it in my life in many different ways: racial abuse, gender abuse. I know what it feels like. And in this situation it was discrimination about my health. She could tell me that there was something wrong with me, but that the wrong was too hard for her! That's discrimination. I am not able to change something about myself that is inherently *me*.

What was the next step in your healing?

Well *that* was a pretty big one . . . if a psychiatrist was unable to help me then it raised lots of questions about whether I was actually 'sick'. Surely that was her expertise? Her field? I began to question the whole idea of what being 'mentally ill' means; I began to break it down in terms of what it meant to me. At the very beginning it was a relief to be diagnosed, it soothed me somewhat: 'Thank god I'm bipolar! Great . . . manic depression! I'm sick. Look at me. That explains every-thing!' But as I'd gone into what these diagnoses actually were, it just created more questions. I began to wonder whether what was happening to me was a per-fectly normal reaction to events in my life. They now call borderline personality disorder, 'complex trauma', and I like that a lot more; it describes exactly where I have come from.

. . . but I've come to the conclusion that psychiatrists just aren't for me.

Did you find someone who *was* for you?

When I was on the dreadful ward where Laura was, I made a passing comment to one of the nurses as I was leaving: 'So what do I do now? Where do I go now?' She took me aside and suggested a therapist at a mental health clinic, but warned me that he was really confronting. I called him up. The first appointment I started to tell him about my childhood experiences and he waved his hand and said, 'Not interested. Tell me what is happening in your life *now*.' I was immediately offended. But that was a defining moment. Up until that point I had no idea what confronting was; I had no idea how dishonest I had been with myself; I had no idea how to be honest with myself until that first meeting.

At first I could only go every couple of weeks. I couldn't *bear* to be with him, because I couldn't bear to be with myself . . . because that's all it was when I went to him. It felt like he was holding up a mirror for me. But I was also empowered in a way that matters. Psychiatrists at the clinic might have given me different strategies to try, but those strategies were merely *external* techniques and *external* empowerment. The real empowerment that came from him, was that I was allowed to say the things I really felt and really thought without being judged and without feeling that I had to qualify anything. It was *all* okay. It felt as though there was a mutual understanding of my situation. It was a complete sense of freedom around my own choices and my own decisions, the biggest thing being suicide . . . somebody saying to me, 'I would support whatever it is that you've got to do.' That was a defining moment . . . 'Oh my god, this is the ultimate about someone giving a shit about my life.'

So he was saying that your decision, even if that was suicide, was the right one for you.

Yeah! Just giving me the freedom to have those thoughts. My whole life had been about squashing anything that didn't fit in: not showing I was in pain, not showing that I was thirsty, not showing that I needed to breathe . . . all with a nice smile. This was the ultimate. Through my relationship with him I now have an experience of trusting, of being trusted, of respect . . . it was probably the first completely honest relationship I'd had with anybody.

What did he actually do that has allowed you to begin to experience those things?

It's not about doing . . . he just *is*. It's his being. It's a kind of acceptance. It's that I am an okay person. It felt as though we were on a spiritual journey and he was learning as much from me as I was from him . . . I'd never had a sense of that before. It was a balanced relationship . . . it was a connection. He said something interesting to me . . . he said, 'As soon as we put the lives of people into the hands of the healers, and take it out of the hands of the psychiatrists, then that's when the healing will begin.' Perhaps then people will start to look at what they're actually saying when they label someone as 'mentally ill'.

How do you define healing?

It's about knowing that there aren't two groups in life. We all have our own stories to tell. We've all got our own journeys. We all have our own experiences and they are *all* valid. There's not somebody who is more valid than me. Just because the way we tell our stories is different, doesn't mean that we are less. The answer is the same: acceptance, belonging, engagement. It's about someone sitting in front of you, who gives a shit.

It's *not* about diagnoses that separate you from everything you know. It's *not* about isolating people even further than they already feel. At the clinic I hear people talking about integrating people with 'mental illness' into society, but by definition of what they have done, they have made that impossible. They label you as 'mentally ill', and then push you back into a society that thinks, 'Oh my god, *"mental illness"*!' There is a basic lack of understanding. In a way I understand murderers, sexual deviants and people who commit dreadful crimes . . . when you're not accepted and you're not believed as a valid human being, it's so easy to carve yourself into that world and just follow it. If society is telling you, you are bad, then you believe it.

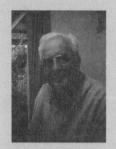

John

John is 74 years old. He is a Deacon in the Anglican Church. *'The German mystic Meister Eckhart wrote that the eternal birth of the Divine Son takes place continuously in each of us. His writing speaks profoundly of my life: before my breakdown I was trying to serve God. Afterwards, God was in me, helping me to do the very ordinary.'*

The start

I think there's some motivation from realising the start.

When I was born I weighed only two pounds. In the 1930s there was no special apparatus for premature babies. That fact speaks very highly of the nursing that was given, but it also says to me that I am fortunate to be alive. To be born under such a circumstance has always made me feel that there was some purpose to my life.

I come from a family that loves music. Dad was secretary to the brass band. I attempted to play the flugel horn, but although I persisted with it for some time, I couldn't pick it up. Eventually I gave up. Although I regretted not being able to fulfil my father's desires for me, it actually freed me up to join the church choir. A Methodist schoolteacher who played the organ in the Church of England (as it was called in those days) was looking for choir boys and so I was taken into that wider family and made 'The Child of God and an Inheritor of the Kingdom of Heaven'. My father's father was a keen churchman, but my parents were not and so I felt it was appropriate that church music should be my first love. If I'd had any aptitude for the flugel horn I wouldn't have been able to follow my schoolteacher's request to join the choir and God would have been non-existent . . . and I wouldn't now be wearing my collar back to front!

You can also see that there has been an ecumenism there since the word go. I was brought into the church by a Methodist, I sang in a Church of England choir, later I worked in the Uniting Church bookshop, and then I started going to a Catholic nun for spiritual direction. Ecumenism comes from a Greek word that means 'house'. It's used to speak of the different Christian denominations. It's the relationship across the board. It's done me good not to just be in my own little box. It's a widening experience in all respects, not just in terms of religion. I view people as being created by God so that they do the things that He would have them do, whether they realise it or not . . . or whether they are believers or not, or whether they are of whatever faith, or whatever culture, or whatever mental capacity . . .

And there's a great interest for me in the meaning of names. My name 'John' means 'God is gracious'. There were no Johns in my family and my paternal grandfather complained about the choice of my name. I recall a Christmas midnight mass when I was a teenager – the words from the prologue of St John's Gospel spoke of John the Baptist, but I felt that they referred to me too:

There came a man, sent from God, whose name was John.

John 1:6

My lifelong calling to the priesthood jumped out of that moment. I've never forgotten it. It hooked me in and on reflecting back on it, I know that I'm called to bless. I have spent my whole life looking forward to the priesthood. That calling has never left me.

I met my wife at an Australian (now Anglican) Board of Missions Conference. The church brought us together. We were married in 1956. I had to set aside my calling because of lack of support from my parents and also a lack of the funds that my parish priest said I would need in order to put myself through theological college. I couldn't afford it. I didn't have that privilege. I suppose at the back of all of this is the money side of things. You have to do what you can with what you've got.

I needed to have an occupation to earn money to support a family and so I chose insurance. My wife and I moved to the city and in 1962 I finished my General Insurance exams. To be a priest I had to have a degree so in the same year I started to study Theology. A friend of mine studied part-time and so I just modelled myself on him. I studied and attended tutorials after work as well as coping with two young children, a son and a daughter.

Not having the kind of brain that absorbs things, it was a lot of effort and I had to work like crazy just to scrape through. There were so many different subjects to cover. I was going pretty smoothly for about six years . . .

In any case I got right up to my optional subject. I tried to do Greek but had no aptitude at all, so I had to do an alternate subject and I picked Ethics. And Ethics knocked me around like crazy. One of the things we had to look at was the Nuremburg War Trials that were brought by the Allies against members of the German services after World War Two. Those tried could not use the defence that 'my boss told me to do it, there-fore it exonerates me of responsibility'. I think it is the dilemma of all the services. When a side is victorious they can try the other lot even though they work under the same principles. It threw me into the really hard part of life. It made me wonder, if there *was* a God then why were all these terrible things happening? I suppose it weakened my faith. I was also tired and out of my depth and I began to blame . . . to blame my parents for not supporting me, blame the parish priest for not making things easier and I began to blame God for all the troubles and perversions of the world.

Do you remember the film *A Beautiful Mind* about the mathematician John Nash? I remember watching a TV program on him in which he makes a remark about how he worked for years to achieve his goal and how the pressure built as he got near the end point of what he was doing. That was so true for me too.

. . . and so you can imagine that I was right at my last subject, looking at all these horrible things and also having in the back of my mind the pressure of 'what's going to happen next?' And that was simply too much for me. I cracked. I went under. And I went under three times and it took an awful long while before life was really worth living again.

Cracked

I remember going down the backyard at the place I lived and I think there was moonlight . . . I remember the moonlight . . . and I now know damn well where the word 'lunatic' comes from . . . 'moon' in Latin is *luna*! It was a peculiar sort of light. It was unreal and it set me off in a way . . . The other day I was reading something about The Buddha and the story spoke of moonlight and I thought, 'Oh *yeah*?'

In any case, I was on a fantastic and unreal high and I

never wanted it to change. I wanted to live on that high forever. I was rushing around, trying to do everything so quickly. But I was behaving stupidly. Abnormally. I was trying to prove that there was nothing wrong with me. Eventually my wife took me to the doctor, and she gave me an injection just to calm things down a bit. She sent me to the first of three psychiatrists. From 1970 on, I was mentally sick, on and off, for many years.

You mention that high. Was there also a corresponding low?

Yes. And also a terrible anger that had lain dormant for years. But overall I recall a state of non-being and divine absence. I felt as though I was no longer a person. I felt useless. I had all the time in the world, but I didn't have the *capacity* to do a darn thing. I couldn't even concentrate to read books or grasp information. It was just so difficult. And my confidence was shot to bits. I suppose from a Christian perspective 'confidence' is '*confide*-ence' in God but there was no *confiding* in God because he just didn't exist any more.

I was working for the AMP Society at the time and they were very good to me. They knew what was going on and they were okay with that. They paid my salary so that we could keep the home fires burning so to speak.

You didn't feel the need to hide the fact of your illness?

I've never tried to hide that I've had breakdowns and things. I don't think there's any point in that. It's part of who I am.

And people are receptive to that?

It doesn't worry them.

But I think in its own way that job contributed to my illness. I had initially worked for a much smaller

Australian company and my speciality had been accident insurance. When AMP took the company over, they accepted me as well. It was a big company and I hadn't worked for a big company before. They put me into Life/New Business and I had to check life insurance policies. I had to compare a strip of typing against the proposal and then sign it. That's what I had to do for years. Can you imagine anything more boring than that? There was never any joy out of doing that! I'd gone from a job that had a lot of variety to just this one boring sort of situation.

But I can't really remember much about the feelings of those times, except that there was no future. There was only a grave, a big pit, and there was nothing else.

A grave?

Yes. The grave symbolised an everlasting nothingness. A huge amount of emptiness. The loss of confidence in God came about through that experience of emptiness. There was nothing there. I remember once hearing of a carpenter who said that he thought people were 'like shavings, pieces of wood wrapped around emptiness'. That was so true for me too.

When I started to write things up I also connected my state of health with Jesus' cry on the cross.

Could you explain that connection more fully?

Well, it was just a cry of desperation. The whole thing.

My God, my God, why have you forsaken me?
Matthew 27:46

I felt so alone. I felt nobody understood me. I had always been a very happy person, I had started off with all these high aspirations, but now I was completely lost . . . and

I didn't think that I would ever be well again . . . it was bleak. Everything was bleak and in the end, when it was over, I was just so thankful that I could do very ordinary things.

At the time one of my friends told me that nobody would ever want to employ me. I guess he was saying it with the best of intentions. Undoubtedly he could see implications in mental illness where that could be the case and he thought I should prepare myself for that sort of rebuff . . . but it didn't do me a whole lot of good to hear it.

You mentioned that you saw three psychiatrists.

With the first man I had rapport. I related to him immediately.

There was a connection?

Yes. There was a connection and that was *most* important. He was a practising Roman Catholic so there was an affinity of one Christian to another, which meant a lot to me . . . and it was just the attitude of the man.

Did the fact that he was a practising Christian help you to reconnect with divinity in some way?

That's probably putting words in my mouth. What was important to me was the relationship. I had somebody I could speak to. It broke through my isolation. You can't speak to your friends because they don't know what you're on about. They can sympathise with you if you have broken an arm or lost a leg, but when your mind goes, that's a different kettle of fish altogether and it scares people. They don't know how to approach you.

Apart from that first injection, were you put on medication?

I started off with something that was meant to slow me down and so it affected my capacity to think. I wanted to be able to think through the situation I was in and therefore I didn't want to take it. I was throwing the pills over the back fence and doing all sorts of crazy things with them. But in the end I found that I *had* to take them because I *needed* to be slowed down. I can't remember taking much else.

Eventually I went back to work. But then I went under again. I suspect I was still frustrated and not fully healed. I liken the whole situation to drowning . . . where you go under three times. Unfortunately the first psychiatrist (who had lectured at the university) needed to conform to new government regulations and obtain Australian degrees, so he was not available this time. With the second psychiatrist I had no affinity. He didn't have any knowledge of the Christian experience and I suppose this was necessary in order to understand me and connect with me. I've no doubt that he was a good psychiatrist but I recognised from this episode, that if you go to a psychiatrist, it's the *need to relate* that's most important . . . that's what matters.

But then there was another period when I was alright for a while, and then when I went under *again*, I was referred to the third psychiatrist. He sent me to a private hospital – I must have needed to be confined there and I suspect my wife would have needed the break. But overall he was quite good. He was dealing with all these miserable people and yet he was so obviously happy. His cheerfulness hooked me in.

And as things turned out he must have helped considerably. After seeing him I had an experience that changed everything . . . the ground firmed up beneath my feet.

The ground
Can you remember the details of that experience?

I can remember exactly . . . I was walking back to

work one lunchtime along the front of the National Australia Bank and I simply felt that the ground beneath my feet was *firm*. It was amazing. It was amazing! It was just instantaneous. It was a feeling of something solid at last. It was the feeling of seeing land after being at sea for a long time. It would be strange to call it a conversion experience, because it was just so ordinary . . . but from that point on things gradually improved.

Was there something specific that brought about this experience?

No. Do you know the German mystic Meister Eckhart? He was a thirteenth-century German mystic . . . he said that instead of God out *there* in heaven, he's in *here* . . . God's in *us*. Eckhart wanted to get rid of the perception that God was living on some cloud up in the sky. And that's also the message of the fourth gospel . . . John's gospel. It's *that* message that makes John's gospel different to the other three. God is not separate. God is not a commodity. He is part of you.

I also think of David Helfgott in the movie *Shine*, who said that it was music that broke him and music that made him. My life is a parallel. It's theology that broke me and theology that made me.

Are you saying that you see the whole process of your illness as one of realising that instead of God being outside of you, God was actually within?

Indeed. I would not be without that. That's my Being. Amazingly enough, I'm more myself than I've ever been.

How had you related to God before your breakdown?

Possibly in a normal way for any run-of-the-mill Anglican. Before my breakdown I was trying to serve God. Afterwards, God was in me, helping me to do the very ordinary. It was a complete change of outlook.

Did the understanding that God was within come about that particular day?

No. It's just gradually come over the years. It was taking Eckhart into my heart through my own experience. There's nothing known about him really . . . about his private life, but I think he must have had similar sorts of experiences to those I've been through, because he believed that to achieve great things in life, it might first be necessary to stumble or break down in some way. Eckhart was also in charge of all the Dominican Houses in Europe so he was a busy chap; he wasn't just some hermit or ascetic sitting all alone in contemplation with nothing much to do.

Apart from the ground becoming firm beneath your feet and your overall vision of the meaning of your illness, were there more specific factors that contributed to becoming well?

On reflection there were actually four components to my being well. Two came before I was ill and two during my illness.

The first was Ainslie Meares' book, *The Door of Serenity*. It's about Meares' treatment of a schizophrenic patient, Jennifer, and the paintings through which she tried to communicate with him. I had read that book *before* becoming ill and it had been the first time I had come across anything like that. There was such a depth to it. It became one of the major reasons for my determination to be well. I thought, 'well if she can get better perhaps I can too'. It was a motivation. It was something in the back of my mind.

I suppose I also found hope in a person being mad and being treated with so much care that she got well. This is a quote from that book:

These are great days. I felt that I had penetrated the barrier. I was through the barrier of insanity . . . To the observer it must have appeared that the patient was talking rubbish to me and I was talking rubbish to the patient. This was so on the face of it, yet the rubbish we were talking was full of meaning.

The situation was crowded with paradoxes. Jennifer had been unable to speak to me because she was mad. Now it seemed to me that it had only been my sanity which had prevented me from conversing with Jennifer.

Now, when I ignored all ideas of sane conversation, I could talk with her, within the limits of our vocabulary, in the language of symbolism.

I also had in my possession a letter that Father Ian Herring had written to Ainslie Meares after reading this book. He wrote:

> It would appear that Jennifer's pilgrimage to sanity is a faithful expression of the classical redemptive pilgrimage of a soul in hell to the freedom of heaven.

I related to Jennifer.

The second thing that happened prior to my illness was that I had read Theology to a blind man. He was an amazing bloke. I heard that he wanted someone to read to him and so I'd read to him. He'd have the text put on to a tape recorder and that's how he studied. He was already a lawyer and then he studied Theology and passed that too.

What did he give you in terms of getting well?

Like Jennifer he gave me motivation. I thought that if he could overcome his affliction, I could get better too. And he also gave me persistence. He taught me that you don't just take a disability lying down, you do something about it. He could deal with his blindness and still be such a remarkable and cheerful man. He had the sharpest sense of humour I've ever known. If you asked him if he wanted tea or coffee, he'd answer, 'Yes.' You learnt never to ask a 'double question' because his *yes* was inevitably a Clayton's answer.

And what were the significant components to your wellness that came during your illness?

The first was Christ's cry on the cross, which I mentioned earlier. Christ thought of his personality as being one with God, and I believe it was the first time in his life that he felt utterly abandoned. It was as though in making that cry my own I was joined to that of my Lord and it became one of restoring faith and bringing healing.

The second was the scripture passage from St Paul's letter to the Romans (8.28):

> . . . all things work together for good for those who love
> God, to those who are are called according to his purpose.

Martin Luther used to say that the letter to the Romans was his bread and butter. And out of the bread and butter jumps that bit. It means so much. It was a possibility that there was hope.

And that suffering has a purpose?

Suffering is a gift . . . and to recognise that gift, truly takes you into the heart of God.

My discovery that many of the great spiritual writers – including Mother Teresa of Calcutta – say that suffering is a gift was a great joy to me . . . it hit me between the eyes! It makes it so much easier to accept the road that I've travelled down. Suffering can seem to be so negative yet it can, if we allow it, produce in our Being the positive gift of compassion. Compassion doesn't come out of thin air.

Compassion

Compassion can grow from suffering?

Having gone through hell, you can relate . . . you can more readily imagine what people are going through. For instance, one of our parishioners had a daughter living interstate with a three-month-old baby, and this daughter committed suicide because she felt that she couldn't care for the baby adequately. She obviously had postnatal depression. I went and saw the grandmother and we could speak about things quite openly because we had both been through hell . . . well she was going through hell at that moment. You feel you can talk to people. You're not shy about coming forward. You get into hard situations and you feel that there's no need to back off. You can be as caring as you can for others. It's a capacity to be there for people.

In another instance, I was at a service in the cathedral that's held once a month. The music comes from the community of Taize in southern France. It has a type of plainsong flavour about it . . . it's a bit different . . . it's very popular with younger people. The point is that people come up to you for prayer for what's troubling them. A woman came up to me and said, 'I don't think I can ever be happy again.' And I dived into my own experience and I remembered Our Lord's cry from the Cross. It had meant such a very positive thing for me. And so I asked that woman to make that cry her own, hoping in the back of my mind that it would be a situation where she could be rescued – the same as I had been.

Of all the attributes of God, I think compassion is the most vital. And I believe that this is where the church has to change. That's the big challenge of the moment . . . to be a compassionate church.

How would the church as a whole express that compassion?

Serving people rather than being something in themselves.

Do you think the modern church has it wrong?

No. Compassion has always been an ideal of the church. It stems from the injunction to love God and your neighbour. But I believe that if we are to 'see with God's eyes' (seeing as God does), I think the vision needs to be wider than it is now. I believe that in the modern world it is necessary to see that people of great leadership and religious insight arise in *many* cultures. There are also people who care, who are of no particular faith.

The emphasis needs to change from the head to the heart, and to accommodate this vision the *whole* of humanity should reach its compassionate potential. The church cannot confine compassion any more than it can stop the Creator working through a wider creation. Compassion is the tool that in the end will defeat terrorism and the slowness of capitalist nations to respond to disasters. Its thrust should be not to defeat negative activity but continually improve on the positive.

I would think that most people go to church to be good or to be helped to be made good . . . there is not enough emphasis on helping people really relate to others who need help . . . though I believe this is changing.

How would you help people to relate to others?

By encouragement. In his book *A Spirituality Named Compassion and the Healing of the Global Village, Humpty Dumpty and Us*, Matthew Fox, a Dominican priest and spiritual theologian says that to en-*cour*-age relates to the heart – 'heart' in French is *couer*. You're encouraging people to grow, to get out of their own selfish centres and try to be something more.

To bless

I assume by relating those experiences of compassion from your own life, that you *did* eventually get back to your study of Theology?

In 1981 I attempted to finish my diploma. You can imagine the difficulty in trying to get back to my studies after such a long time! I stayed clear of Ethics though and chose Christian Education instead. The pass mark was 50 and I got 46, and so I had to do *another* year.

But my health continued to improve and then in 1982, twenty years after beginning, I completed my studies. I passed my Diploma in Theology. This helped me to get the job of theological book buyer at the Uniting Church Bookshop. I was in that job seven years and I just loved it. It was *me*. I used to think that if I couldn't be a minister myself at least I could help others become ministers. I knew the need for books while you were studying.

In 1990 the bookshop closed. It was a blow in many ways, especially financially, and to this day it remains my last paid full-time employment.

In June the same year I was made a deacon, some 40 years after knowing I was called.

Do you wish to continue until you are a priest?

Yes! I've always wished to continue. Even at the age of 74! The calling I had as a teenager was a calling to *bless*. That's how I know in my own mind that I'm called to be a priest and not a deacon like I am at the moment. A priest can bless but a deacon can't.

What does 'to bless' actually mean?

The blessing is at the end of the service. A blessing bestows the gift of the Peace of God.

What is necessary for you to become a priest?

It needs the approval of the current bishop. If he doesn't want to, he doesn't have to. That's all it is. My Diploma of Theology is enough education to become a priest.

So it's up to one person?

It's all up to what he thinks . . . and you can't appeal against it. You can't do anything about it.

Is your amount of service taken into account?

Well I've got a huge amount of service . . . I think I don't fit his pattern of education. You need to go to college and follow through with certain things he thinks are essential . . . in other words, I'm probably a little too home-spun for him.

Time

I was appointed to a parish to help the priest while he was waiting for a heart transplant. The heart didn't come. I then worked with his successor and we made a good team.

When I started taking funerals, one of the readings that this priest used was Ecclesiastes 3:1–8:

1 For everything there is a season,
   and a time for every purpose under heaven;
2 a time to be born, and a time to die;
   a time to plant, and a time to pluck up that which
   is planted;
3 a time to kill, and a time to heal;
   a time to break down, and a time to build up;
4 a time to weep, and a time to laugh;
   a time to mourn, and a time to dance;

5   a time to cast away stones, and a time to gather
    stones together;
    a time to embrace, and a time to refrain from embracing;
6   a time to seek, and a time to lose;
    a time to keep, and a time to cast away;
7   a time to tear, and a time to sew;
    a time to keep silence, and a time to speak;
8   a time to love, and a time to hate;
    a time for war, and a time for peace.

Albert Nolan, a priest of the Dominican order in South Africa who wrote a book called *Jesus Before Christianity*, believes you can't interpret scripture without knowing how Our Lord would have interpreted *time*.

Time in this sense is not chronological or quantitative as in our Western way of thinking. Rather it's thematic and qualitative; it's the quality of what is happening in your experience. It also contains within it paradoxes that relate to Eckhart's work. To think in Eckhart's way of paradox is to hold the opposites in tension, so that both parts are necessary in life. (These paradoxes can also refer to the Yin and Yang of Chinese philosophy.)

Seeing time in this way has been a major breakthrough for me and I feel that it has enormous relevance to my episodes of illness. For instance, Verse 3, 'A time to break down, and a time to build up' could be applied to *health* instead of the obvious application to building. Verse 4, 'A time to weep, and a time to laugh' also means a great deal to me, because when I was sick I had no sense of humour.

In this light I also think it is interesting to consider the current situation in Iraq. I wonder whether Adolf Hitler was not stopped because it was *a time for war*. It would be very easy for us to wish that this was not so, but the fact is that *the time for right action* was not taken to stop him. Perhaps Iraq now poses a similar question.

What time is it, in this, our day?

Health

Only recently a piece of roughness took me by surprise.

I was over at the local library and they were having a sale of books and one in particular took my eye, *The Holy Blood and the Holy Grail* by Michael Baigent. I believe that this is where Dan Brown got a lot of his ideas for *The Da Vinci Code*. As I was reading *The Da Vinci Code* I could say to myself that it was just a novel and therefore the way he handled the Christian tradition didn't worry me. But when I picked *this* book up, I started to get interested in the way the author had written, thought and researched; I started to go along with it. He was saying that Our Lord escaped his crucifixion and that the Holy Blood was his bloodline and that therefore it was an hereditary thing. It puts a totally different perspective on everything. I started to wonder, 'Oh God, have I wasted all my years?' And that's not an easy thing to consider.

But I started to think about it and after a while I realised that this need not worry me. I am well now, and all those things that seemed to have, on reflection, some purpose, no historian could bugger up! My spiritual reality is more important than anything an historian might write about; no historian can ever take away my experiences. It was important to look at this and consider it, but it was more important to come to the conclusion that it can't touch me.

Somebody asked me why I hadn't left it alone. I couldn't. It left me on a limb for a little while but I knew I had to find a way through it.

So even though your are now well, life doesn't always run smoothly!

Exactly. Life continually changes. It is a struggle and it is a joy.

What do you feel is the essence of health?

To my mind health means having a wideness to see the good in people. You don't need to shine yourself, to appreciate what others are like.

I read somewhere, one of the Russian writers, who said that humility comes from the Latin word *humus* which means 'to grow' – it's an earthy thing. It's got nothing to do with a false sort of sponginess or artificiality . . .

You also see growth as part of health?

Yes. Growing is an essential part of my Being. When I saw the Archbishop about being priested once, he asked me why I wanted to be a priest. I answered, 'So I can grow.' He said, 'That's got nothing to do with it.' But I think he was very wrong. I think it's got everything to do with it.

Do you see that process of growth continuing?

Yes. You don't stop. It's a continual challenge to be as Christ was and is.

I recently did a service at a nearby retirement home and I focused on six people for whom I felt this was the ultimate purpose or focus of their life. To my mind they are some of the giants of their various ages and cultures. In each of them I could see a quality that I also felt was in Christ. They didn't just talk about God they actually embodied the *presence* of God. It was about the Divine Word or *logos* as it was made incarnate. It is these people we need to emulate today if religion is to be rescued from terrorism overseas or sex scandals at home.

Wisdom

Menahem Nahum, a Kievan Russian visionary and reformer of Judaism who lived in eighteenth century Chernobyl. He wrote in times of great hardship (the Russians persecuted the Jews) and yet he was a visionary with a very wide outlook. He was a guy who could see God in everything. He saw wisdom in *all* of creation. He felt that the wisdom of God took on the form of everything that is in existence. That's the wisdom the world needs right now.

Forgiveness

Nelson Mandela, the South African politician, who to me embodies forgiveness. He put forgiveness into practice because he worked with his enemies in order to establish a better world. I believe that without forgiveness, freedom is not attainable. I also remember that he wrote lovingly of his wife after their divorce. He *must* have been able to forgive to write so lovingly of her!

I also believe that it is no accident that the first words Christ says from the cross are 'Father forgive them, for they don't know what they are doing'. (Luke 23:34). He was rejected by his townspeople at Nazareth, then he was crucified – which was one of the most terrible forms of torture – and all he did was to think of other people! It's incredible! I think the fact that his first words are about forgiveness is just vital. I don't think he could have uttered those words in such a stressful situation if forgiveness was not a prime principle *throughout* his life.

We tend to think of forgiveness as something we do inwardly, rather than something we do outwardly . . . asking for forgiveness for *others*. I think if there is *anyone* who remains unforgiven then there will be deep within the offended one something which binds and captures.

Persistence

Siddhartha (The Buddha) who lived two-and-a-half millennia ago, I believe embodies persistence. Once alone on his travels he came to a beautiful spot by the banks of a flowing river, and there made a resolution to sit and not rise again until he had reached enlightenment.

Compassion

Mary McKillop the nineteenth-century Australian nun who I believe embodied compassion and indeed *emphasises* the continuing need for compassion within the church. She wished to care for the poor *wherever* she saw a need, not just within her own diocese. She believed in her work and would not abandon her ideals even when excommunicated by the bishop for not wanting to conform. (Interestingly, on his deathbed the same bishop reinstated her . . . even bishops have guilty consciences!)

Joy

Tjilbruke the Adelaide Plains Aborigine from the Dreamtime. Tjilbruke sorrowed over the ritual slaying of his young relative who had broken a tribal law. When carrying his relative for burial, at every place he stopped a spring (of tears) welled up. After his sorrowful journey Tjilbruke was transformed into an ibis. I believe this points to the fact that deep sadness gives way to deep joy.

At my very first clergy conference in 1990 we were taken by bus to the Tjilbruke Memorial at Kingston Park in Adelaide. We were told Tjilbruke's story by an Aboriginal man. At the very moment he mentioned Tjilbruke's transformation into an ibis, I looked up in the sky and the sunlight shone on the white wings of an ibis! I'll never forget it.

Unity

Mechtild of Magdeburg, the thirteenth-century German, who was for most of her long, active adult life, a Beguine. The Beguines were often a threat to those in power. They were condemned and then not condemned by the Pope. They were welcomed and then driven out by the bishops.

It was *such* a joy to discover her writing on unity; her idea that the Divine is truly in us and can *never* be taken from us under any circumstances. She believed that the bond with the Divine is so strong that it is as though we are fused together and poured into a single mould. We can *never* be separated from the Creator.

This is where I find my health . . .

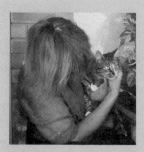

Linda

Linda is 47 years old. She is an extremely creative person and enjoys working with both her hands and her mind. She works on a voluntary basis with the Salvation Army and values the interactions it brings. She would like to help others go through life more easily than she has. *'This is a photo of me holding one of my cats. My cats are my lifeline. They're my children. I have five cats and a little dog that is now blind. They keep me alive and I am indebted to them for that.'*

I've been searching for help for nineteen years. I have visited countless psychiatrists. I always brought up the fact that my problems started in my childhood. I wanted to bring it out into the open but none of them have been interested in what happened. I don't even have all the recollections myself. The psychs have all been aware of that, but none of them have been prepared to do anything about it. They offer me a pill and tell me to go home. 'Don't think and don't feel' is their motto. I had no one to turn to then and I have no one to turn to now. It keeps coming back to being that little child . . . I mourn for this little girl inside me.

What can you tell me about that child?

I was number three of four children. My brothers hated me. My sister who was four years older didn't play with me. I was always the good girl who feared being hurt.

Physical abuse?

Not for myself. My eldest brother was bashed for spilling sugar for instance. My parents hated him. My sister suffered from epilepsy so she was a second-class citizen in their eyes and was emotionally abused as a result. I didn't want to be part of it. I chose to stay out of trouble and be the A-grade student and 'the understanding one'. They had their drunken parties and I'd be the one who made hors d'oeuvres. I went without so the others could have things. But whatever I achieved or did was never good enough. I did everything for love and attention and I never got it. I felt I was in the way.

At school I felt like a fraud. I acted like a normal person but I knew that I wasn't. Other children had families that baked biscuits and went on outings together. We had none of that. A trip to the beach would have to last us for two years. Every day I feared coming home from school. Christmas was awful. I was ashamed of my life. I'd make up stories or not let anyone in. And no one ever knew.

My parents were of a European background and were a product of their time. They went through the Second World War and suffered horrific things. Mum was raped at gunpoint by German soldiers. But they chose to deal with it by drinking themselves into oblivion for most of their lives. They gave no thought as to how it affected us children.

How *did* it affect you?

It had a major impact. I think it was one of the reasons I was molested as a child. Mum was never there. Nor was Dad. They didn't protect me. There were times we'd all get ready to go out, but we'd only get as far as their drunken friends in the city. We'd be given ten shillings to go and wander the streets all day and all night. Four young children. And this happened often. Everything revolved around alcohol and we didn't come into the picture.

Even when I was molested as a child, I'm not sure it occurred to me to tell Mum about it. When I was in my twenties, visions came to me of what had happened. I discussed them with my mother then, but she dismissed the incident because the perpetrator was seventeen or eighteen and 'only a boy'. The fact that I might have been five, six or seven at the time, didn't come into it. It didn't occur to her that it might have any affect on me. I could never go to her for anything. Ever.

And it's carried into my whole adult life. I still feel like an alien. So often I say, 'Beam me up, Scotty! I don't want to be here any more. I've had enough.' I don't fit in. When I am with people I feel like I'm a fraud. I can't be me. In fact I don't even know who 'me' is any more because I've spent my whole life trying to please everyone else. I've got to be the perfect person. Everyone can use and abuse me but I have no right to stand up, say what I think, be emotional . . . none of it. People say I am a strong woman, but inside I am so vulnerable and weak that in a blink, I'm gone.

What do you mean by 'gone'?

I struggle every day with staying alive.

It was only in my late twenties when I read a book called *Toxic Parents* by Susan Forward that I realised my life had all been bullshit. I related to that book so much that I felt it had been written for me. It tore me apart because I had never dared to question anything. Who was I to question? I didn't have questions. I was too frightened. And *now* I have so many questions and I want answers. And that's what I struggle with. There are just so many questions.

What was it that the book said?

It said I was a person after all and that I *did* count. The book said that as the number three child I was the invisible child . . . and that's how I've felt my whole life: *invisible*. I've lived my whole life on the outside looking in. Even as I'm talking to you, another part of me is actually standing behind watching *us* having a conversation. I'm not really here. I'm standing over *there* watching the whole scene.

It also had something about parents who were alcoholics. Seeing it in black and white like that had such an impact. It took so long to come to terms with the book . . . it brought up such pain. The pain was indescribable; it felt like it was coming out of my pores. And anger. But although I was very angry, I didn't share what I had read with my parents. I continued to push it all away. There was an incident when my brother assaulted me and I got the blame. Although my parents had seen my brother punch me in the head with his fist and I went to the police, they weren't prepared to back me up. An argument ensued from that, and I used it as my escape point. I felt I then had a reason, in *their* eyes, not to come back any more. I stopped seeing my parents for three years so that I didn't have to think about it any more. But the real reason was that they failed me miserably. I was robbed of my childhood. And then I just felt guilt: guilt about being molested as a child, guilt about everything I do . . .

They still don't know to this day how they have affected me. None of them do.

Have you tried to tell them?

No.

Do they know of the struggles you've been through?

No. In their minds I'm over-emotional. I'm a loser. They see my need for medication as pill-popping . . .

I had an abortion at fifteen. I was looking for love.

Mum dropped me off at the hospital because she was too embarrassed to come in with me. For years after, she would lecture me, 'God is punishing me for murdering your child. I signed that piece of paper!' She threw that at me for years. I pushed that pain away too. More guilt. More guilt. As a child I even thought I should have been able to stop the man who molested me. Everything is my fault.

You mentioned that when you had the abortion you were looking for love . . .

The only love I've ever felt is from my children and my pets. Unconditional love that is. I love my daughters to bits. My daughter says to me, 'You're not just my mum any more, you're also my best friend.' I don't see them just as my children, I see them as my friends as well. For that reason I have respect for them . . . even though I have failed them in the past and still do.

But otherwise I don't know what love is, not even from my husband. All I feel comfortable with is abuse. That's why I married the guy I married. He abused me emotionally. I don't give nice guys a second look. I even have days now when I just want someone to hurt me . . .

Why?

When I'm abused it reinforces that I'm just a piece of shit after all, and it's a relief. My brother once said to me, 'Stop being a victim.' I'll stop being a victim when people stop putting shit on me.

What do you mean by 'being a victim'?

Allowing others to have control over me . . . but I had no other way. Some days I just can't stand myself. I can't even be in the same room as myself . . . and that's when I start to lose control. I feel it coming. I feel it building. It's like a dark hole. I warn the doctors.

Is it triggered by something in particular?

It's in me the whole time. There doesn't need to be a trigger. I might just wake up feeling that way and it intensifies as the day goes on. I try to push the bad talk away. There is a person inside who abuses me, a man, and he'll always win. That's why sometimes I become reclusive. I don't want to walk out the door. I don't want people looking at me. I don't want to look at them.

And what happens as that process builds?

I want to be swallowed up by the earth. Disappear. I look for a way to kill myself. I overdose on medication. I had a near-death experience once and I found out for myself what the meaning of life is . . .

Which is . . . ?

Basically the meaning of life is that 'this is it'. I don't believe in religion any more, nor the afterlife, reincarnation, God . . . all of that is out the window. I have to question that now . . . the revelation as I was dying was, *this is it*. We've only got one chance and this is it. We die and that's the end of the story. You're dead. You're gone.

What has that knowing brought to your life?

Live now. There are no excuses. Take responsibility now. It all just *is*. I knew with every bit of me that that was the truth . . . but still, I pushed it to the side for quite some time, because doctors, friends, everyone discounted it. Who do you tell anything to?

Nobody wanted to listen?

No. All I'm trying to do in my life is enlighten others about mental health and about sexual abuse. My main principle in life is: 'If you don't like it done to yourself, don't do it to others.' I even quoted some statistics to my psychiatrist the other day: one in three women have been sexually abused at some point in their life. She said she thought it was closer to 50 per cent . . . I mean, who reports it? And as far as mental health system goes, I have a conspiracy theory – not really – that they're all just trying to shut us up with antidepressants. Everyone I know is either on them, or is supposed to be on them . . . from fifteen-year-olds to my mother at 80. It's about quietening everyone down: 'Don't have emotions! Don't you dare stick up for yourself!'

Do you feel they're trying to narrow everyone to a certain level of behaviour?

Yes. Like they did years ago. So many women were put on tranquilisers. How over-medicated was the population 30 or 40 years ago? Now it's antidepressants.

They're really just reinforcing that it is okay to control someone. Everyone else has had their turn at controlling my life and now they are doing the same. I never felt I had a right to be me and by giving me drugs they're just reinforcing that.

You mentioned at the beginning of the interview that you'd been searching for help for nineteen years. At what point in your life did you first seek help?

I had a car accident in '86. I nearly miscarried. My marriage broke down. Even though I couldn't stand my husband, I felt like such a failure. I felt so inadequate. I wasn't sure how I could bring up my children on my own. 'I can't even change a fuse, so what use am I to anyone?' My whole world was falling apart, I wasn't coping and so I sought out psychiatric help. And that was the beginning.

My psychiatrist *did* help me through that period, but he gave me medication . . . and I doubled my weight within six months . . . and so I threw all my pills and tablets in the bin. But then when he moved interstate I had to see others . . .

And that's when I got involved in the public mental

health system. I moved on to other antidepressants, tranquilisers and really strong painkillers for my osteoarthritis. I was over-medicated. I was having so many side effects that they ended up giving me medications to counteract the side effects! I was taking 30 or 40 pills a day and it was out of hand. But now because I've become 'borderline personality disorder', they can't offer me medications any more. They've given up.

When were you told you had borderline personality disorder?

Approximately three years ago was the first time I heard those words. Nobody explained it to me. It was as though they made up the label on the spot. Even though I showed symptoms of bipolar disorder (mania and depression), they didn't seem to think I had that. Apparently because of my overdose attempts – my death wish – I have borderline personality disorder. I found out later that the disorder usually begins from childhood trauma, like the sexual abuse and the taunting and humiliation I suffered from my brothers.

What do the words 'borderline personality disorder' mean for you?

Not a lot. It's as though it's their way of putting me into the 'too hard basket'. The whole time it's been, 'It's too hard, we don't know how to treat you, so go home.' They'll treat me if I overdose, but as soon as they've treated me, I'm out the door. I'll get no help because they can't control my overdosing or my death wish with medication.

In the public system, I could access a psychiatrist once every three months, and I remember once, on my second visit, the psychiatrist saying, 'You need more intensive help than we can offer you, so there's no point in you coming.' He was virtually saying that *no* help was better than *some* help! He was telling me that there was no help for me. They just assumed I would go away.

Years ago I got involved with a psych hospital attached to a local hospital. I don't remember how I got involved . . . I was detained once. Other times I went voluntarily.

Why were you detained?

I told the psychiatrist that I was so depressed that not only did I want to gas myself, I also wanted to gas my children. I didn't mean that I was going to do it or intended to do it, I was simply saying that I had thought about it a week or so earlier. I was trying to demonstrate the intensity of what I was feeling. But she detained me on the spot and my kids went into foster care.

The psychiatrist didn't acknowledge the depths of your depression?

No. And it only made the depression worse. Much worse. And then my kids were indeed put into a position in which they weren't safe. They still have nightmares about it. I have always had such difficulty verbalising my feelings and here I was simply telling the psychiatrist the truth. I was looking for help and all I got was locked up. I was punished for being honest. And all I learnt from that incident was not to open my mouth. I am very careful now about what I say to those who have the power to detain me.

And what happens when you go into a psych hospital? You're left on your own! There's no one to talk to. The nurses are too busy. There are no psychs on hand. There's no one on hand unless you make an appointment, and that might be once a week.

So what *did* happen during your time in hospital?

Nothing! They'd medicate you and that was it. They'd just wait until it was time to send you home. We were left to our own devices. We weren't allowed to go to our rooms. We were bored shitless, smoked a lot and talked. It was all of us, the so-called 'mentally ill', who were the therapy. We did our own therapy by talking with one another. And that happened every time when I went to other psych hospitals too, whether it was years ago or recently.

The only time they actually *did* talk to me was in another local hospital when I was there for two days in intensive care and then had thirteen days of detention. Then there was help available. Psychs were on hand. They were able to tell me about borderline . . . but still the therapy you get is from being mates. There was friendship, frankness, openness, honesty, sharing. They may have given us different labels, but we were all still *people*! We respected each other as human beings. Once you are labelled 'mentally ill' people are scared of you. It becomes us and them, and I'm tired of that. The media portray the 'mentally ill' as violent. But the truth is that we'd much rather kill *ourselves* than anybody else. I apologise to an ant or a spider if I kill it. I don't want to hurt anybody or anything.

But generally when I turn up at hospital, if I am too intense with my feelings, then I feel they make me wait longer. Last time I was there, they didn't treat me for six hours. Some of the nurses who don't know my disorder seemed angry with me. They didn't want to treat me. They gave me 'the look'. They judged me because I'm a psych patient. They looked at me with disdain, as though I had no right to be there. And that only added to my distress. I go there to be safe. But I suppose the fact is that they're not actually trained to deal with the 'mentally ill' and only rarely do they have psych nurses on hand. Perhaps the answer is for more nurses to be trained. But where are the resources? It seems that all they do is close more wards . . . they're going backwards.

And the crisis service is hopeless too. One time I rang them in distress. I had all my tablets on the table, I'd been boozing and was ready to overdose. I was thinking, 'But I really don't want to do this.' And I rang this guy up and asked him to help talk me out of overdosing. He wouldn't do it, because he was more interested in the fact that he had to knock off in ten minutes. He said, 'If you feel you need to overdose, well that's what you need to do.' And that's what I did.

I haven't found any help in the system. Where are we supposed to go? Just disappear? Sometimes it seems as though they *want* us all to commit suicide. It's like there is no room for me if I can't be like everyone else. And what does that say about our society? Not a lot.

In an ideal world how would you envisage a system that would really help?

I need help to try to understand who I am. The answer is within but I need guidance for that. I want to be treated as if I am a fellow human being and not a patient. I want someone who sits and talks with me and doesn't talk down to me. I don't get that in the system. It's like *they're* the experts and they have all the answers. It's as though *I* know nothing. I'd like to become articulate enough to teach others how to put things into words so that psychiatrists and the system *will* listen . . . when people feel stuff strongly it's really hard for them to find the right words or portray the intensity of what is going on.

But I think it all boils down to the fact that I believe I'm not worth anything. And no amount of medication or therapy can change that; no amount of someone telling me that I am beautiful or that I am worthy. I have always needed guidance and someone who is prepared to talk with me about the childhood sexual abuse. I have always been ready to talk about it, but no one else ever was . . . I was always aware of that little girl crying for help and no one ever listening. However, in the past few months I've begun to see a counsellor who specialises in sexual abuse. She's the first person to whom I have been able to say specifically what happened . . . but it's going to take years of unravelling and I'm not sure that I've got the strength to do that.

You mentioned earlier that you felt the answer was within.

Yes. We've got it all inside ourselves. My belief is that we don't need help from psychiatrists or religion. People choose pills or God because they can't believe in themselves. I do respect that people choose those paths to help them get through life, but I choose to try to learn to believe in myself instead. And love myself . . . because if I don't love myself, how on earth can anyone else? All our answers are inside but we don't know how to access them. I am so passionate about people having spirit, creativity, talent . . .

What do you think that spirit is?

Your soul perhaps. Your self. Your inner being.

So even though you don't believe in God or reincarnation or religion, you still believe there is something that could be called a soul?

Yes. But only while I'm here on earth. While I'm on earth there is a soul within . . . a being within . . . it's not a soul that carries through to another life. It's what I am in *this* life. Now. Somewhere along the line people want to squash that . . . the person who molested me, my parents, my husband, the system . . . although they can never snuff out my fundamental spirit, they do everything in their power to try to take it away. They just want to take and take and take. And it hurts more than any physical pain. Emotional abuse is far worse than physical abuse. And then my anger just turns inwards and then I'm the one who's guilty again. I'm guilty of all the world's wrongs.

How does that fundamental spirit make its presence felt in your life?

It's partly about listening to my instincts. If I listen to my instincts well then I am right 100 per cent of the time, but I've been taught not to do that!

In what situations might you listen to your instincts?

Anything! It might be simply putting a glass vase somewhere and knowing that if I leave it there it will break and then following my instincts to move it. Sometimes I can know how people are going to behave. I'm only learning again who I am because I've been too busy trying to please everyone so that they'll love me. I'm such a perfectionist that twelve out of ten is not good enough. I can't reach a goal any more because they're unreachable.

What do you feel you have to be perfect about?

Everything. I like being creative — crafts, baking, making chocolates and biscuits at Christmas time. I far outdo anything that any chocolate company could do — the way I present them, the way I make them, the way they taste . . . they're perfect. But I'm so embarrassed! I can't take the compliments. I fear the success as much as I fear the failure and so I sabotage everything I do. I'm *never* going to be a winner. Perhaps I have to accept that in my own eyes, I'm never going to be a winner. I just get more and more confused about who I am . . .

In those instances when you might move a glass

vase and you know that that was the right thing for you to do, do you get a sense then of who you are?

When it happens, yeah! It's like, 'You *did* know! See! There you go!' Sometimes when I predict something will happen and it does, I do think, 'Well I knew it, because I *listened* to myself!' Even driving the car I have begun to *feel* when I drive. I *feel* what is happening around me much more. I'm learning to trust myself and trust what I'm feeling.

Do you feel that down that path is who you are?

Yeah, perhaps. But I'm still not sure. I know I want to contribute somehow in life. I want to give back some of what I've learnt by getting through horrendous situations that others may not have gone through. But as soon as I say that, I start to think I'm a fraud again. That I'm not strong . . . and then I want to give up . . . In a couple of weeks I'm going for an appointment with a plastic surgeon. I have such an issue with the way I look. I've lost all the weight I put on when I was taking antidepressants . . . I didn't lose the weight for any personal reasons, only the fact that I didn't want to be made fun of when I was lying dead on a slab in the morgue. But now I have all this flabby skin and I am disgusted. I won't have sex with a man. I want love and I want to have a relationship but I feel that I'm not good enough. And I am sure that I won't be accepted for surgery, and I know that then I'll find myself questioning why I am alive again.

When I go into these dark tunnels and get swallowed by self-loathing and hatred . . . even the fact that I have two wonderful children and all these cats to take care of . . . it all flies out the window. And then I can't access any of the knowledge, logic and strategies I have learnt. When I start to feel bad, I've learnt to distract myself for instance – to go for a walk and stick to it. But when I go into the tunnel, then it's all gone. And then I have to die. I can't be here any more. Just let me die! And then I overdose . . . and then when I've crossed the line, I realise that I really don't want to die at all . . . and then I seek help . . . What do I want? . . .

What *do* you want?

I just want to be that little girl . . . loved . . . I want to know what my role in life is . . . and I want a rest. I want a rest from life. In a way that's the main value of detox or a psych hospital – it's a holiday away from your problems. You can detach yourself from your life. You can feel that you're in a safe little cave for a while.

So the idea of a retreat is an important one?

Yes. That would be the answer. Even if it was just for a weekend.

What would that give you?

Freedom. Freedom to be myself. I wouldn't have to put on the persona that I do every day. I could be myself. *Myself.* I wouldn't have to pretend to be anyone else. I long for solitude in my everyday life, but then when I'm by myself I fear that I will die.

You mentioned earlier that you were seeing a counsellor who specialises in sexual abuse.

Well it has been hard work on my own, but I now have a support system that I have set up with the help of one particular GP who specialises in mood disorders. I now have a counsellor who helps me with sexual abuse, a psychiatrist and a psychologist who gives me the guidance I need.

What does that 'guidance' mean as opposed to what you have been offered in the mental health system?

Guidance is helping me to find my way. It is recognising that there are paths that I can go down. It is a way to live and to survive. I don't necessarily talk about the personal problems with the psychologist. It's about life and strategies to cope. For instance, I need to be taught how to react in certain situations. But it's also about enlightening me . . . he's my teacher. He is my *life* teacher. He has taught me about listening to myself and not being afraid to feel.

I knew about stuff like instinct before, but he has validated that. He has validated all the stuff that I've felt over all the years but never been able to put into words – like the sense of that spirit inside. And the fact that in that spirit is true knowledge. Knowledge doesn't come from your ego or your mind. All our answers are within, but there is no one out there to show us how to access it.

But above all he's given me validation – the fact that I feel a certain way because it is true. I remember he once read me the first bit from M. Scott Peck's book, *The Road Less Travelled*. It said, 'Life's difficult'. I thought, 'Shit yeah!' It was that validation that life *really* is difficult that was so important. Once I accepted that life as a whole actually *was* difficult, then life was no longer quite as difficult. Being seen and being heard is so important. I've started the process of reporting the sexual abuse that happened to me when I was young. I don't need the molester to be charged or any of that – it's just so important to see it all written down in black and white.

And what has the psychiatrist given you?

She's been very helpful, but I've only seen her twice.

And what do get from the sexual abuse counsellor that you don't get from the psychologist or the psychiatrist?

She's like a shoulder to cry on. Sometimes that's what I need. Other times I'm not receptive to that. If I go to my psychologist, I know that I'm not going to get a shoulder to cry on, because he makes me stand on my own two feet and be responsible for who I am and for every word that comes out of my mouth. I can also tell the sexual abuse counsellor the personal and more intimate things – things I haven't been able to share with anyone in my whole life.

Is that because she works primarily with sexual abuse?

No. It's just her as a person. I trust her and so I'm not scared to open up to her. With her it's the personal relationship that is important . . . you don't get that sense of personal relationship in the mental health system.

Do you feel you are beginning to move ahead?

No.

Can you imagine a time when you might be able to?

That's certainly my intention. I *want* to live. I want to teach myself how to get through these crises. When I'm in distress, it's like I'm screaming on the inside. It's like, 'Why can't anyone else hear it?' My head feels like it's going to explode. There's no one listening.

So the psychologist and the counsellor don't listen to that screaming?

The psychologist, no. I don't think I've made him aware of the intensity of my distress, because I fear that I'd be a failure then. I feel I have to show him a strong face, that I am a strong woman – that I'm not weak and vulnerable. The sexual abuse counsellor has heard me more than anyone else has. She's felt my pain. She's recognised that I am in pain and that it is okay to be in pain. I think that's what we need to learn: not to be frightened of the pain, not to push it aside and put on a happy face. That's what psychiatry tells you: 'Don't have emotions', 'Don't feel that you have the right to stand up for yourself', 'Don't be a person!'

So that's what you feel the system is telling you – don't be a person.

Yes. They all want me to go away because I don't fit. That's when they medicate you.

Are you on medication at the moment?

I stopped medication a few weeks ago. I was on the main antidepressant of the moment. They increased the dosage and all that did was make me sweat. They brought the dosage down again and it did nothing. I still had the bad times. So I thought, 'Why the hell am I poisoning myself with this stuff if it is having no effect?' All I get from the psychiatrists is, 'Well if you don't want to take it, then how do you expect us to help you?' That's all the feedback. Either you take the drug or you can fuck off. And that's all I've had, all along.

Medication for me isn't the answer. It's just a bandaid that never solves anything. That's where the mental health system goes wrong ... they're just giving us bandaids and nobody wants to know the cause: How did you get here? Why did you get here? Sometimes I think that realistically it might be better if I die; it seems the logical step to take..

Even with the support system you have now set up, do you still feel you won't make it?

It's still not enough. Ultimately I still have to do all the work myself. There is still such self-loathing there, so that it seems pointless to do it. I end up sabotaging everything. It's all too much. But for other people I think that is the road to go down: belief in the self. And that's what I want to make a point of in this interview: *don't believe in anybody but yourself.* If I had started down that

road twenty years ago it would have made a big difference. I can see that that's the way.

But now I am tired. The mountain is so high that
I'm never going to get to the top. I am physically and
emotionally tired.

I suspect that I'm not going to make it and that's
okay.

Christie

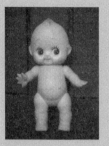

Christie is 32 years old. She has been diagnosed with bipolar disorder, anxiety disorder and major depression. *'This photo is of a Kewpie doll. I remember a lot of happy times as a kid with my Kewpie doll. She came everywhere with me, even in the bath. I didn't keep the original one but a good friend knew that I liked them and found this one in an op-shop for me.'*

To look good

I'll start with my childhood . . .

My parents split up when I was five. My mum found out that my dad was having quite a few affairs. They tried to sort it out but they couldn't. Then at some point my dad left. My mum was only about 28 at the time and she definitely felt alone and scared raising two kids without my dad.

There was another family living down the road, Elizabeth and Mick and their two boys. We were friendly with them and went to parties there. At some point after my dad left, my mum started seeing Mick down the road. He eventually left his wife for my mum . . . and I don't know how it happened, but after that my dad ended up marrying Elizabeth. They basically swapped partners.

I do know that Mum and Elizabeth had started to end their friendship before Mum started seeing Mick. There was a side to her that Mum didn't like very much. At one point before my parents split up, my father had gone to America and Mum took us to Melbourne. Elizabeth thought Mum was avoiding her and was

197

actually still in the house. Elizabeth came to the house, turned off the electricity and broke into the house. We came home and there was blood everywhere because she had cut herself when she broke the window. She had some pretty irrational tendencies! When Mum ended up with her husband she wasn't too happy.

From the time I was about seven, Elizabeth was my stepmother and my brother and I went there every weekend. She was just . . . manipulative. She'd buy us gifts and then tell us we were ungrateful and bad and then take them away. Almost every weekend we would get a lecture about something. She would always tell us things Mum got up to. Her and Dad were always fighting. It was very aggressive. Very violent. At one stage she wanted her two boys to start calling my father 'Dad'. So they sat us down and asked if that was okay with us. My brother and I were too scared to say the wrong thing, so we just said, 'Yes, that's fine.' But then we were in trouble for saying 'yes' because we shouldn't have wanted someone else to call our father 'Dad'. We were put into catch-22 situations. As kids we couldn't really work out what was going on. We were just trying to avoid conflict. I remember one night when they came over to pick us up and she started calling Mum a 'fucking cunt' in front of us.

I've since learnt that she has a background too. Her childhood wasn't great and she obviously learnt destructive ways of dealing with her problems. But although I've got an understanding now about where she was at . . . to do that to children! . . . I would never do that to children, regardless of the situation. And she still does it to this day.

The other side of things . . . at home with Mum and my stepdad . . . we weren't really a family. My brother and I would come home and we'd be put in one room to watch television and they'd sit in another room and watch television. There was a real separation. I didn't really like my stepdad much, but at least, unlike my stepmother, he was predictable and I knew where I stood.

When I was about thirteen my father and stepmother moved interstate. I was really relieved that I didn't have to go there any more.

The main thing I learnt from all of this was that I had to say the right thing and please people all the time. I'd try to work out what people were thinking, what they wanted me to say or what they wanted me to do.

As I got older this became worse. It got deeper and deeper and deeper. I compared myself to other people: 'Is that girl prettier than me? . . . Is she better than me?' I was trying hard all the time to impress people and get them to like me. If people liked me, I felt safe. I tried to be the perfect weight and get the perfect job. I didn't realise that some of these things weren't things that I wanted to do simply because I was *not* allowed to make mistakes. Instead of learning from my mistakes, I'd just turn around and try harder to do the same thing over and over . . . but when you do that you eventually break down. The following quote is from GROW's[9] little blue book:

> If I want at all costs to look good, I am living to please or impress others, and I am an alienated and worldly individual.[10]

---

9   GROW is a worldwide community mental health movement started in Sydney in 1957.

10   GROW program, *The Program of Growth to Maturity* (the little blue book), copyright © GROW INTERNATIONAL, A.C.T., Australia, 2005, p.17.

The little blue book contains all of the GROW program and it's what we use in our meetings. The little blue book was put together by a group of people who recovered from mental breakdown and recorded what worked for them. It's been added to since then and it still gets added to now. It can seem a bit weird when you first come into GROW because the language is a bit old-fashioned. I think it could be adjusted to fit better with the times. But the main thing is to work on the book with others. You've got to be in a group and interpret it together.

Anyway, it was a big shock to me when I first read that quote about looking good. It's pretty harsh because as a kid I couldn't have done any different; that's how I learnt to survive. I didn't have any other way to cope. But it wasn't really reading it in the book that led me to understand how much I wanted to please and impress others. Rather, someone else in GROW said to me, 'Look, this is the problem I have, I think it may be your problem too.' The main thing about GROW is that you meet real friends who tell you the truth.

I started to observe my behaviour and realised that I always changed to whatever environment I was in. We all do that to some extent; you're different at a party than you are at a board meeting. But what I was doing was radical change. I was like a performer . . . and the anxiety that produced in me was just enormous . . . the anxiety was there all the time.

I didn't really know who I was. Ever.

To be at home
I went to university and studied marketing. I didn't even know what marketing was. I just studied it because that's what everyone else was doing. It was a career in

which you made money and impressed people.

I'd had boyfriends throughout high school but at uni I met a guy called Steve and I just loved him to death. He treated me well and I started to feel a bit secure.

But after about three years things got rough. He smoked a lot of pot, took acid and was a small-time drug dealer. He certainly wasn't big time or anything and it didn't seem like a big deal to me; he just sold it to his mates. I never had the attitude that he was a bad person for doing drugs. Anyway he got caught growing plants at his place and then came to live with me. At that stage I was living with my brother, who was just starting out in his career in alcoholism. The whole situation got too stressful for me.

Around this time I had also started to experiment with drugs (ecstasy and acid), but didn't take them to the extent that Steve did. Most of the people I knew were doing it and I just wanted to see what it was like. It was a recreational, fun thing to do. I wish to make that point that although I don't do drugs now, because I realise it's not a good thing to do, I don't think it was a either a consequence of or contributing factor to my mental suffering at that time. It was the events that were difficult for me to deal with.

Added to the situation was another guy who was showing interest in me. He *looked* a lot better than Steve did. Steve was a bit of a hippy with long hair and this guy had a nice car, classic good looks, ambition and financial promise . . . eventually I just left Steve for this other guy. I didn't have any insight into the fact that I'd left something that *was* good for something that *looked* good.

After about a month I started to get depressed. I started to miss Steve and all his friends. I realised that I'd made a huge mistake. I was sure that if there was a God, he wasn't ever going to forgive me. I thought I had only one chance in my life and I'd used it up. I thought I would never meet anyone like Steve ever again. I thought that I'd made my bed and now I had to lie in it.

I got more and more depressed but felt too weak to leave this guy. There came a time when I had to move out of where I was living, and he did too, and so we thought the obvious thing was to move in together. During the time we were actually shifting I had my first breakdown. I walked into a supermarket and I was trying to make a distinction between two cleaning products and I had my first anxiety attack. It was like a rush of electricity going through my body. I couldn't see properly. Voices were fading in and out. The supermarket was spinning around. And I thought, 'I'm dying. I'm having a heart attack! Something's really wrong.' It wasn't like anything I had ever experienced. I somehow got through the checkout and drove to my mum's. I said, 'Mum there's something really really wrong with me.' I was just so scared.

And then I started having panic attacks one after the other. Over and over. I was vomiting and I completely lost the plot. There was also an accompanying feeling of *homesickness*. I was going into something that was wrong and I was homesick for something that felt right. I remember having that same feeling of homesickness when I was little. There was a time Dad wanted to have us for six weeks during the school holidays. After being there for a week and contemplating another five . . . I was found wandering around at five o'clock in the morning, wanting to go home to my mum's.

GROW talks about our three vital needs:

To be SOMEONE – Unique Identity and Personal Value
To be AT HOME – Security and Loving Harmony
To be GOING SOMEWHERE – Purpose and Progress[11]

Security and loving harmony were continually taken away from me because they were never in *me*. I always looked for them in particular situations. I'd never developed them *inside* because as a kid I'd never had them from my parents.

That was the big thing: *I didn't feel at home.*

The hopelessness of it all

I went to see a GP. She said I had major depression and gave me antidepressants. She said the panic attacks were as a result of the depression. I knew someone who had suffered from postnatal depression and I tried to tell the doctor that what I was going through seemed pretty similar. She dismissed me like I was being a silly little girl.

I rang an association that specialised in panic and anxiety. They supported me and put me on to a psychologist. He tried to hypnotise me and also did lots of visualisation stuff. He'd get me to put my problems onto a leaf and watch them float away. None of that stuff ever worked with me. I told him a bit about my background but he didn't seem to think that it was anything unusual. His specialisation was childhood sexual abuse and in the end he just said, 'Look I can't work out what's wrong with you. I can't help you.' So I still felt I was weak . . . and felt I wasn't trying hard enough.

Even my friends . . . not one of them ever said, 'That's

---

11   ibid., p.13

bad or odd.' I never got the impression from anyone that my childhood was at all disturbing or something that I could have problems from later on in life. People said, 'You've got no reason to be like this.' As a result I also told myself that it had nothing to do with my childhood. And that made me even more anxious, more depressed . . . I read lots of self-help books on depression, inner life . . . I tried meditation . . . I even tried to meditate *perfectly* . . . I'd spend ages trying to get the mantras just right . . . but nothing had a lasting impact . . . but I probably tried too hard . . .

I kept going to work even though I continued to have panic attacks there. Luckily my boss was pretty sympathetic. Also, because I'd developed an enormous amount of self-control by needing to look good all the time, I could still go forward and do all the things I had to do. I tried to forget about my feelings and eventually things started to get a bit better.

I left the guy and was okay for a while, but after that I really lost the plot again. Anxiety. Panic attacks. I was suicidal *all* the time. I thought I was the worst person in the world. I had trouble doing things. I was chronically afraid throughout the day. I didn't sleep. When I'd occasionally have a day or two of feeling okay, I'd really hope that it would last.

The mum and dad of a school friend offered to let me live with them for a while. I had my security and loving harmony back again but nothing really changed *inside*. I still had the idea that I had to do everything alone because otherwise I was weak. I also didn't know how I could ever show my gratitude to them (related to being told I was ungrateful and having presents taken away). I got sick again when I was living with them and that was just the worst of the worst.

There were all these people saying, 'It's okay, we accept you have a mental illness.' But I still felt I was just the weakest person. 'I've got all this support and I *still* can't do it.'

I kept thinking that I had to get back to the way I was before it all happened. I got sick at 21 and I kept thinking I had to be like I was before that. I had no concept of change and moving forward within myself, my life and my relationships. I had no concept of change as an ongoing process. I only ever thought of moving forward in a financial sense: getting a good job, getting a bigger and bigger house, getting more and more material possessions.

The only thing that *did* seem to work a little were massive changes of scene. I moved interstate to live with my father for a while, I moved in and out with guys, I got jobs here and there . . . I really think these changes were my own little version of shock treatment . . . the improvement would last for a week and then I'd be back to how I was.

> God doesn't usually change things. He mostly changes people so that they can change things.[12]

I saw another psychiatrist who just talked about medication and said, 'You're a beautiful, smart woman. Go and meet some good-looking wealthy man, get a job, and you'll be fine.' That wasn't helpful at all because it fitted right in with all the superficial beliefs I'd had in the first place.

It only added to the hopelessness of it all.

---

12   ibid., p.21

Cracking life

I got a job and met a beautiful woman who had a similar background to me . . . but she also had some insight into it. She knew how her childhood had affected her. She also told me great things about myself: that I *truly* was intelligent, beautiful and talented. She also liked the same sort of movies. We became pretty much inseparable.

After I'd got sick I'd read that I shouldn't be taking drugs with my condition, so in my attempt to be perfect, I hadn't taken them for years and years. But after I met this woman I started doing it again as a fun thing. We started going out to nightclubs and I started taking ecstasy and smoking pot. This time however, rather than just doing it on the weekends I was also doing it through the week. And I just got higher and higher and higher . . . and then I had my first manic episode. I thought I'd finally cracked life . . . I thought I'd never be depressed again. I thought I was *well*! Looking back I think the mania was the result of the combination of the drugs and finally meeting a person who understood me. I was over-confident. I was flying.

One night we were out nightclubbing and I met an old friend from school called Andrew. He'd had a problem with heroin and he told me that his two best mates had died from heroin overdoses. I liked him and felt for him but I didn't really want to get involved with a 'heroin addict'. I continued to get higher and higher and about a month later I ran into him again. I had certain risk-taking behaviours associated with the mania and went around to his house and fell in love with him. Within three weeks I'd moved him into my place . . . and that's when things started to go bad. He was still scoring . . . we ran my credit card up to $5000 ... we got evicted ... and then I started to go down ... I ended up in hospital. I was just so depressed and suicidal. A lot of people close to me blamed Andrew and didn't understand how I could be with him. They thought he was just a junkie with no moral values. It was total confusion. The doctors suggested ECT.

I guess the ECT did what it was supposed do, because it wiped out about two months of my life. I couldn't remember anything and if I did, it was like it had happened to somebody else. It was like a visualisation of a movie. There were no feelings associated with anything, which is probably what I needed. A lot of people had turned their back on me and the only one who seemed to care was Andrew. He visited me every day in hospital and said he was praying for me. Because of the ECT, when I came out, I couldn't even remember how to drive to my mum's place ... it was pretty scary. I wouldn't recommend it to anyone ... but it did block out the pain.

I was discharged from the psychiatric ward. I had nowhere to live and I was feeling pretty desperate about it. A guy who was on the ward with me offered to let me live at his place. He had some pretty huge problems, but because I was so desperate for somewhere to live, I moved in with him. It didn't work out at all. If I'd been well I would have realised that his intention was to have a relationship with me. It was then that someone from GROW called Doug told me that I could live at his place until I got back on my feet.

At that time I'd been going to a few GROW meetings, but hadn't really taken it on all that seriously. In fact, when I first came into GROW my anxiety had only worsened. I thought I was *really* at the bottom of the heap.

Going to a psychiatrist was okay, but going to GROW was *so* bad. I thought it was full of all these people who had *really* lost the plot. But I kept going to the groups and they kept helping me with my thinking, giving me tasks to do and they affirmed me for it.

The meaning of life

I had always had all these searching questions about the meaning of life but I'd just never asked them or when I did ask them, people would say, 'You think too much, that's your problem.' They were questions like: What's really important? What happens after we die? How can all these bad things be happening in the world? Doug seemed to have answers and he had worked it out through coming to GROW. It wasn't like he was saying he had all the answers but after talking with him I began to see the value of GROW.

I met another guy in GROW called Darryl and he also seemed to have some pretty good answers to my questions. But most of all, it was the way that he could think about things and make decisions that made a big impression on me. He'd weigh things up and give himself the time to think. I began to slow down my thinking and really *really* think about something, rather than thinking that I had to come up with the right answer straight away. I learnt that the world wasn't divided up into rights and wrongs. I learnt to question absolutes.

After a while I began to see many things differently. One of the things GROW says is, 'Emphasise what *is*, rather than what *isn't*'.[13] At first when I started to do that it felt a bit like Louise Hay's pie-in-the-sky stuff.

---

13 ibid., p.18

It didn't go down well with me. But things did start to change. I remember going to a Grower's house. Normally I would have walked in and thought, 'Oh it's *so* seventies. The carpet's not a nice colour.' I would have been an expert at looking at things in the house and finding fault with them. But I'd practised GROW's advice so much that I started to zoom in on other things: rosary beads hanging on the wall, art work. Personal things and relationships became more important. All the other stuff started to fade out.

GROW's Principle of Personal Value says we just have to have belief in persons to get well. It says that all human beings are basically of the same value no matter what our abilities, our talents or what we look like. We all have the same value.

> . . . this Principle is a radically levelling one, inasmuch as it requires anyone who sincerely believes it to be true of himself, to go on and affirm it of any and every other human being . . .[14]

I guess in my situation, I could see value in other people, but I didn't believe it of myself. Eventually I had to turn it around and say, 'Well if it's in other people, then it has to be in me as well. If I can believe that the person in front of me *can* improve and *is* improving, I have to believe it about myself.' I also started to realise that a relationship with people is the most important thing in life. I think that's how we work out who we are. It's through deep relationships with others that we begin to get a sense of ourselves. It's not through all the shallow crap that goes on out there. But having

---

14 ibid., p.69

said that, although I love people I also like to be on my own. I need a bit of both in my life.

Relationships have also given me strength, particularly in dealing with conflict. In the past I tried to avoid conflict all the time. I've got one friend called Patrice who shows strength when dealing with conflict and sometimes now, when a conflict situation comes up, it's almost like I can hear her very matter-of-fact words in my head: 'Stick up for yourself!' If I have to ask my boss for something, I hear her words, 'Just ask him!'

There's also a lot of stuff in GROW about being ordinary. It's about telling the truth. It's about learning to tell people how I feel and realising that they're not going to dislike me for it. 'Ordinary' doesn't mean average or normal. Being ordinary is just being myself and doing ordinary things. Eating healthy food is ordinary. Sitting with a group of people and having a cup of coffee without having to build myself up is ordinary. It's about not being of lesser value or greater value. It's also how I work out whether to try something new or not. For example, Andrew wanted to go swimming and I'd only ever wanted to do aerobics and nothing else. He'd ask, 'Why don't you come swimming?' Normally I would have said no because I'd get anxious and worry whether I'd be able to do it, so now I say to myself, 'Well it's a pretty ordinary thing to go swimming. Why don't I just do it and see what it feels like? I might enjoy it.'

My social experiences before GROW had usually been centred around going to pubs and drinking, so coming into a group and being in a community setting was very important for me. I started to make *real* friends. I used to have a panicky little voice inside, 'Poor me. I'm too scared to do that. I'll get hurt,' which was followed by whipping myself, 'You *can* you stupid weakling.'

Because I've made real friends in GROW, I've been able to treat myself like that too. It's like there are friends inside me now. There's an adult side to me now.

I'm beginning to find out who I am.

Where the truth is

I hadn't grown up with God and I'd never been to church. I believed that if there was a 'power' of some sort, it would be just like my dad and stepmum and punish me for my mistakes. GROW says that there are four views of God and that as we mature our view of God changes.

1. The Overall Power is Impersonal or Evil.
2. God is a Severe Taskmaster and Judge.
3. God is a Kind Saviour, Healer and Teacher.
4. God is a Supreme Friend and Lover.[15]

For a long time I fluctuated between the first and second views of God, especially when I made a mistake. Then God was like a Taskmaster and I'd think, 'You've just got to try harder Christie! You're a stupid weakling.'

It was through GROW's Principle of Personal Value that it became possible for me to walk into a church and begin to talk to Christians with interest and open-mindedness. Until then I'd always been anti-Christian. I'd hated Christians. They were so happy that I thought they were just kidding themselves. But GROW itself isn't any denomination or faith and not all people who come to GROW believe in God. The blue book makes this clear:

For sheer willingness to help in human suffering the vital difference is clearly not between religious believers and

---

15 ibid., pp.73–74

unbelievers but between those who care and those who don't care. . . .

That is why, though GROW is profoundly spiritual and God-centred, it can draw no clear line between believers and unbelievers; and some unbelievers make far better Growers, and better friends for growth, than some believers.[16]

But I've eventually come to Christianity, both through GROW and my partner, Andrew. I think Christianity is where the truth is.

From the first day I met him, Andrew was a Christian. Even though he went off the tracks and was into heroin, he knows it's the truth. He started talking with me about Christianity. He started me reading the Bible. I could find fault with a lot of it but I kept reading it anyway.

I'd always thought the story of Jesus Christ was a fable. I hadn't realised he was a real person. And it was the fact that he was a real person and could understand how people really felt that appealed to me. He hung out with prostitutes and he stood up to the Pharisees. He stood up for the truth. He had compassion for other people. He had forgiveness.

Forgiveness is important to me because it means that I can make a mistake and it's okay. I might make it again and I might make it a third time, but if I don't forgive myself for it, I'll work myself into a hole. Because of eternal life, there's also a sense that life isn't a race. I'm not going to run out of time. I always thought I had to accumulate things or get a job because otherwise I would run out of time. I have also realised that all my worries and little things aren't really all that important any more. I still feel them but they don't become a

---

16 ibid., p.22

part of me any more. I don't let my thinking go with those feelings.

I'm only just starting to understand that Christianity is a relationship with Christ. That relationship means that instead of worrying I talk to Christ now. That's been a huge help. I tell Him how I'm feeling, I tell Him that I know He's there and that He can look after things. It's comforting and it's secure. I feel at home. It's like He knows me. If I'm wondering what to do about something, I always think about what He may have done. But when I have no control over a situation and I feel really really stuck I can say, 'I can't do anything as a person so I'll leave it in your hands.'

With Christianity and Christ I've got something good to build my life on. It's a foundation for me. A foundation for building who I am. When I'm making plans for my future, I've now got a base of what's important.

Growing

One day, Andrew and I were walking our dog on the beach. We were both a bit down in the dumps with only a few days of work here and there. We were wondering where we were going. I said to him, 'If we want to pursue this Christian thing, we're going to have to start going to church and get into a community.' (We'd been looking for a church and had been to a few, but they hadn't really suited us. They were mostly filled with old people.) With that our dog ran over to another dog to say hello. It was with a man who was in his seventies. We said hello. He asked us how we were and at first I said, 'Well thanks.' But then I said, 'Actually we're not that well really, we're both a bit depressed . . .' And we got into a conversation. I wondered why we were saying all this stuff to a stranger. I told him that we were thinking we should start going to church. And he said, 'Well I'm actually a retired Uniting Church minister.' I said, 'You're joking!' From that day on he started coming up to our place every Tuesday night for Bible study. Last week two more young people came along who have just become interested in Christianity and are outside the life of the church. So my faith is growing.

Growth is an ongoing process. It is about getting closer to God and becoming as much like him as we possibly can. It's about the qualities of His that I embody. I know that I'm a patient person. I know that I have a good heart. I also have compassion for people. I've always had compassion but I never really recognised it as a good thing and I never really realised that not everyone has it.

In the past I had always thought I would get it all right one day and arrive somewhere so that I could sit back, relax and everything would be okay. But I don't think life is like that at all. I think life's more of an adventure. Surprises always come along. But the difference now is that my mind is much more open than it used to be and so I have the ability to make a lot more choices . . . but there's still a long way to go.

The most important thing I've learnt is that I am a unique person. I used to have no sense of self and felt like I was a ship at sea that got tossed and turned with the tides. But I've come to realise that it's not all down to fate. I have an inner ability to create who I am. I can work on myself and become who I want to be. That knowledge gives me a much greater sense of purpose and a much greater sense of security. And a depth. I feel like I've got depth to my character now.

Not perfect, yet forgiven.

Patrick

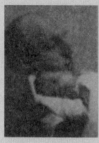

Patrick is 52 years old. He was born in Ireland and moved to Australia at the age of eighteen. He runs a non-profit organisation, Change of Habit. He hopes to take this organisation beyond charity and into humanity. *'I am now happy for the first time in my life. I am happily married. I have a very supportive wife and a beautiful young daughter, both of whom I cherish very much. I also have a little poodle and a very messy bird. My daughter was born thirteen weeks premature. She fought against the odds to be born and to be with us. I was the first human being to hold her. She was so tiny. I watched her struggle for life and I kept thinking, if this little tiny human being can struggle so hard to live, then why am I struggling so hard to die?'*

I first came across something termed 'mental illness' in one of my relatives. She was different from the rest of the family. She was a truly wild Irish woman with long flaming red hair and she was involved in witchcraft. I never saw any goat's heads or black candles around the house, but she did have a cauldron with ladles hanging from the sides and she made little thatched cottages that she put in the garden. I remember in her wildness was an immense creativity and sexuality that even as a small boy I was drawn to. She was true to herself and in that I saw a beauty I didn't see in the rest of my life. But there was also something that scared me. She'd beat up men. Her behaviour could be unpredictable. And every now and then she'd disappear and she'd wind up in a mental institution. I don't know to this present day what she suffered from or indeed if she suffered from something. Perhaps it was simply that she was different. If you are different in our society people automatically assume that there is something wrong with you and so they feel a necessity to put you away for a while.

The part of Ireland in which I grew up was pre-dominantly Catholic. Everyone had very large families. Religious families. Children everywhere. If you were a couple without children people wondered what was wrong with you. You had to have at least half a dozen to a dozen and my family with nine fitted very comfortably into that zone. I was the eldest and I was responsible for looking after all my brothers and sisters and cousins and whoever else was there. I was a bit like the Pied Piper. At the end of the day I could never sleep until everyone was in the house. It was usually my father who came in last. He worked as a barman and I'd hear his whistle in the distance as he came down the street. Only then could I go to sleep . . . but that was the only comfortable and peaceful time I had.

Every day was a battle. It was a fight to survive. Something had happened to my mother. It had to do with the pressures of having an illegitimate child in the 1950s in that sort of Catholic environment. She was ostra-cised. She wanted to put me up for adoption but my grandmother would not allow it. When I was three or four she met and then married my father and he adopted me. But then she started to beat me and I never knew why. I saw such a craziness in her and that craziness scared me. I was never scared of any man as much I was scared of my mother.

Could you describe that craziness a little more?

It was an uncontrollable rage. It was something I saw in her eyes that she always took out on me. Even at an early age I was always wondering 'Well, *what* is wrong with me? What have *I* done wrong?' I got blamed for things that weren't my fault. She took everything as an excuse to beat me. I don't know for sure how my manic depression disorder started but I assume it has its foundations around that time.

Did you first feel the symptoms around that time or did you feel in retrospect that the first seeds were sown then?

The beatings didn't just affect me physically. They affected me sexually as well. At that age, six or seven, I was getting excited from the beatings. And it was the way my body was coping with it. I was getting pleasure from getting beaten. That scared me and confused me. The next time I got a beating I wouldn't exactly say I was looking forward to it but I did know that I now had a way of coping with it. The beatings weren't quite as painful as before. I think somewhere among that smorgasbord of mixed feelings and suffering, pleasure and pain, maybe the seeds of manic depression fell.

How long did the beatings continue?

They went on for a number of years and then they stopped . . . I was eleven perhaps . . . on this particular occasion I knew there was going to be the beating of all beatings . . . because my mother had picked me up from my grandmother's house and walked me along the back lanes between the houses so no one would see her. When we got home no one was there and she just laid into me . . . for no reason. She never needed a reason. When my father came home and asked, 'Where's Patrick?' my mother must have pointed upstairs. I remember him saying, 'Oh God, what has she done this time?' Two doctors came. My shirt was welded to my back with blood and they had to pick the small pieces of shirt out of the blood and welts. And then my grandmother told my mother off and I knew then that it would never happen again. She was exposed.

Then, as a teenager I was involved in the early days of The Troubles – the civil war in Ireland – and it was in this environment that those seeds of manic depression and also alcoholism started to grow. I only knew what was happening around me and it was that same mix of feelings – excitement and fear. I was involved in the violence for about a year, first with just stones and bottles. Then I came across weapons of destruction . . . I remember a friend opening the boot of his car and there lying in front of me was a German Luger and a Thomson machine gun. I knew at that point I had a choice, to get more involved or to get out. I chose to get out. I didn't want to kill anybody. I didn't want to hurt anybody. I could see the potential for risk in situations. I didn't want to die.

I came to Australia. It was a new world and the first thing I felt was *relief*. From responsibility. I didn't have to look after anybody any more. The world was my oyster. I could do what I wanted. It was a wonderful place. And of course, at that time, the first place a young man went to enjoy himself was to the pubs and the bars. I was told I adapted to alcohol with a smile on my face. But apart from that nothing really dramatic was happening. I joined the army for a while in 1971 but was given a medical discharge because I hurt my foot. Eventually I met a girl and we fell in love and got married. At the time I worked as a nursing assistant at a home for intellectually disabled people and I really enjoyed it. It was one of the best jobs I have ever had.

What did you like about it?

Again I liked the exposure to weird and different behaviours. But in this case there was a different label put on it, the label of intellectual disability. And that label said it wasn't their fault . . . simply because that's the way they were born . . . and so society found those people easy to accept. But at home my own behaviour was becoming more and more erratic . . . my son had come along and I didn't want all that responsibility again. I thought, 'Here we go again. I've just left my family behind and now I'm starting my own!' It's hard to describe in a few words, but I would say that I swapped the love of my wife and child for the love of the drink. I walked out on them. But it wasn't a premeditated choice.

What was it that the alcohol offered you?

I loved the stuff. I *loved* the stuff. There is not another word in the English dictionary to describe it. It was a feeling of euphoria. I could take criticism. I could handle pain. But I could also think for myself, and I'd never had the opportunity to do that before. Thinking had always been done for me.

You felt you could be yourself.

I felt I could be Patrick. I felt I could be who I wanted to be. If God has thought of anything better than alcohol I'm sure he's got it up there for himself. When I was drinking I was higher than a 747. I was higher than anything. I would come up with these wonderful stories. I wouldn't need music, thank you very much! I had a wonderful mind for remembering trivial bullshit . . . little passages from the *Reader's Digest*, a repertoire of over 200 jokes . . . I couldn't shut up. There was so much energy there. It came bubbling up out of me like a volcano. I was an entertainer. Everybody loved me.

But for all the good times, I suffered the pain of the down side dreadfully . . . I was exhausted. My body suffered from the lack of sugar in my system. My liver was swollen and painful to touch for about a week afterwards. My head was going crazy, 'Where's my family? Why am I walking around the streets? What's happening to me? Where am I?' The depression lasted as long as I didn't have a drink. And the mania lasted as long as my body could take it.

I just want to say at this point that I don't believe there is such a thing as 'mental illness'. I prefer to call it mental trauma. I think the stigma attached to the words 'mental illness' is too difficult to remove. It becomes embedded in you like a virus and you can't get rid of it. It is like a virus of terminology that society puts on people because they can't find any better words to use.

So you think people who suffer from what is commonly termed 'mental illness' have suffered from some sort of mental trauma.

Absolutely. Everyone suffers from mental trauma, at one time or another. I think the trauma is the beginning of whatever happens. That trauma, whether it be physical or psychological, affects your ability to reason, to cope with ordinary everyday happenings, and to behave like everyone else. When you suffer in your childhood, you can't turn it around and say that it is a chemical imbalance as psychiatry does. Whatever trauma has happened to the mind is like a pattern that leads you to develop more complex issues in dealing with life, like manic depression, like schizophrenia . . .

I remember a nurse in a detox centre was the first human being who gave me some insight into the reasons why I was doing the things I was doing. When I went to that detox I always seemed to have this one particular nurse attending to me. She would feed me and bathe me. In one sense it was very embarrassing because I could do nothing for myself. But one day she asked me if

I had been abused as a child. I was immediately affronted and angry. 'How dare anyone ask me that! Did I have it stamped on my forehead? *Patrick's been abused!*'

Sometime later I'd quietened down and I decided to ask her why she had asked me that question. She replied that over the years she had seen countless men who drank themselves into oblivion, who were completely helpless and hopeless, who could do nothing for themselves, who messed in their pants and couldn't even tie their own shoelaces. And slowly she had realised that like me, they were coming to her as a woman, to have their bodies tended to and washed and cared for in all the ways that a mother should have done when they were children. I remember I just broke down and cried like a baby. It was such a relief. I wasn't mad or crazy. There was actually a reason for it. It all made sense. It was a wonderful feeling. It was the beginning of an opening for me, the beginning of finding who I was. It has taken me many many years since then . . . of drinking and highs and lows . . . but that person who had the time enough to care for me and say what she did . . . she opened a door and said, 'Patrick's in there.'

Beyond the highs and lows, do you see a relationship between the manic depression and the alcoholism?

I think the alcoholism brought the manic depression to a head. I think the sufferings of alcoholism itself, the anti-social behaviour and distortion of my thinking, led me into a full-blown manic depression. I noticed years later that even when I was drinking, I was higher than most people. And I noticed that most people also came down quite easily after a while. When I came down, I came down with an almighty thump and I stayed down there for a long long time . . . until there was another drink to get me up again.

Did you realise at the time that the alcohol was bringing the manic depression to the fore?

No. At that time I didn't realise that the manic depression had hit me. I didn't see what was happening. But there was one incident that really scared me ... when I realised that something was really wrong ... I had a friend I had met at a place for homeless people in Melbourne. His name was Dave and he was much bigger than I was. He was a solid man with big arms who used to be in the police force. Like myself, he'd fallen from grace and I kind of looked after him. We used to do casual work together to get some money for drink. At the time we were working at a football club. One day I went there and Dave wasn't there. I asked the boss, 'Where's Dave? He never misses work. Is he sick?' And he said, 'Oh he's in a hell of a mess. He got hit by a car.' I asked where he was, and the boss said, 'He's heading up the road.' So I ran after him and saw him up ahead of me. I called his name over and over, but he wouldn't turn around. He just kept walking. I kept calling until I got up next to him, and I turned him around and I saw that both his eyes were blackened, his nose was broken, his arm was in a cast ... I said, 'My godfather, what happened to you, Dave? The boss told me you were in a car accident.' And he pulled away from me and kept walking. And I said, 'Dave, what's the matter with you? It's *me*, Patrick!' And he said, 'Don't you remember? *You* did this.' I denied it and he said, 'You were mad. You completely lost the plot. One minute you were just sitting there and the next minute you did this.' I still don't know what happened. Just talking about it now is giving me the shivers. After that I knew that something was definitely wrong with me.

How do you account for that violence now?

I don't think violence is a part of the manic depression. There was something within me, in the combination of the alcoholism and the manic depression. Not all the time. Just every now and then. I think it had something to do with the frustration of trying to understand it all. I think it was the fact of not being able to sit down with someone and discuss what it was like and what was happening to me. I'd been with a few psychiatrists up to this stage and they just put me on medication. There was a Catholic priest who tried to help. He wondered whether something pressing on my brain might be causing the lapses. He thought it would be a good idea if I went to hospital to have it checked out. So I went there and I came back with a smile on my face feeling very important. He asked me what they had said and I told him, 'Well they're going to do a lobotomy on me.' I didn't know what that was. He simply said, 'Over my dead body.' That's the only sort of help that was offered.

Did the lapses continue?

Yes. Sometimes I lost a whole week. Even two weeks. And that went on until I stopped drinking seven years ago. I remember finding myself in hospital in about 1980. I'd been there for a few days with alcohol poisoning. It was about two in the morning and the doctors came to me and asked, 'Have you got anywhere to stay?' and I said, 'No . . . I've got a wife and son somewhere.' But I couldn't really remember. And they said, 'Well you've got no fixed abode then.' I'd heard that phrase before but couldn't really think what it meant. And they said, 'Well don't worry, someone will come and pick you up and they'll take you to a place to stay.' A van from a home for the homeless turned up at the back of the hospital, a man came and asked for me . . . and that was the beginning of the journey for me.

The journey?

The journey that took me into 'mental illness' and alcoholism and living a life that is completely alien to society. A world of every kind of human depravity.

Why do you see that particular point as the beginning?

It was an episode that I could get a handle on. It was a period in my life that I remember reasonably well . . . and I remember clearly the shock the next morning when I woke up . . . of sharing a dormitory with 180 men. All different. Alcoholics. Homeless. 'Mentally ill'. Drug addicts. People who had been recently released from gaol. People with three or four university degrees. People who had been company presidents. Einstein could well have been sleeping next to me . . . And I also remember the mass exodus in the morning. We had to go down and get our clothes from a small room with little pigeon holes. During the night they always fumigated the place . . . a couple of those insect bombs . . . everyone in the area knew where we were from because we smelled of insecticide . . .

Despite the circumstances, you speak of those people with great fondness.

They were wonderful people with all sorts of 'mental illnesses' and I *loved* them all. Those people were my friends. They were my extended family. I still hear their voices. They were the people I felt more comfortable around than the people in society. Yes they were unpredictable. At any time somebody could come up to you and give you a wallop. But that was okay. I *knew* who they were. I wasn't *scared* of them. I wasn't frightened of them. I felt that I was one of them.

For most of my adult life, the people I had been around had been telling me what to do – that I shouldn't be drinking, that I should get a job – they were always trying to direct me where to go. But I didn't want direction. These people just accepted me. There were no questions asked. They didn't care what I'd done. They didn't care where I'd been. They accepted me unconditionally for who I was. I'd never had that feeling before. In many ways I resigned myself to die there. I didn't want to leave. It was as though all these people had come to this castle or this place of utter torture and pain and they had had to leave all their differences, their attitudes, and their pretensions behind them. There was no room for it. I can't paint but I can sculpt a little bit . . . and I can still close my eyes and sculpt the faces of those men. Their characters. Their scars. Through them I can feel their pain. The pain of their fall from grace. And what used to make me angry was *why doesn't someone help them*?

Help them in what way?

Take them aside individually. If society was so powerful, so wonderful, so precious why couldn't they take aside one human being and put every effort into saving them? They ought to be helping individuals . . . say to them, 'Look you've had a nightmare of a journey, now help *me* to help *you* get some quality in your life. Let's help you get out of here. Let's empower you to use the experiences that you've had to make choices so you can have a better quality of life.'

People are under the impression that our lives would be fine if only we could go back to where we came from, but that is an illusion. Society tells you to go back, but you can never go back. I knew a man who was manic depressive like myself, and I heard him singing and playing guitar in the bathroom at a rehab place in

Brisbane . . . and there was a talent competition at a hotel . . . and I entered him in it. I probably shouldn't have done it . . . but all the same, he went through with it and he won. And afterwards he cut his wrists. It was too much for him . . . That's the dilemma. You can't put people back in a society that has ostracised them. So where do you put them? Do you create a new society? A paradise? I don't know . . . I am still so scared of coming back into society, scared of stepping on people's toes.

How long were you homeless for?

About twenty years . . . but I think it's important to make clear that there are different sorts of homelessness. I had always assumed homelessness to mean sleeping rough and being on the streets indefinitely, but you could be sleeping on people's couches, in boarding houses or rooming houses, and still be homeless. Just because you have a roof over your head doesn't mean you have a home. And I also believe there is another side to homelessness that can often lead to the physical side and that is when you don't have a family or anybody who cares for you. And you can also be homeless in your mind or in your spirit. Something could have happened to you as a child that separated you from the trust of someone who was meant to care for you. That is what I believe happened in my case. Homelessness for me started when I separated from my mother . . . when that bond of trust that should have been there, was broken. As a result I could not connect with anybody. And I still feel homeless now. Not until I have bought my own home, a home that no one can take from me, will I feel that I truly have a home.

How did that sense of homelessness in your spirit lead you to a physical homelessness?

I had to follow something in me that I couldn't deny.

It was like a magnet. If I denied it I wouldn't be Patrick. I had to follow something that homelessness is a part of. It was a drive within me that took me to gaols, to rehabilitation clinics, and detox centres. It led me to meet criminals, addicts ... people you would never meet in so-called normal life.

So there was some overarching sense moving you through everything?

Yes. It comes from somewhere in the lower belly section. In the lower abdomen. It is almost like you know something but you don't know what it is. It is a different sort of knowing, like an instinct and you have to follow it. My life would not be worth living if I didn't follow it. But people certainly get hurt in the wake of it. I left my wife without a husband. I left my young son without a father. How can I explain to my son that I left home and became a homeless alcoholic because I was following my instincts? So sometimes I ask if it was all worth it, but I know that I had no choice. It was so strong. Something was happening through me ...

Could you describe in a little more detail the life of which homelessness was a part?

Drinking a lot. Getting into trouble with the police. Getting locked up ... probably 25 or 30 times over the years ... just for a night here and there ... but also for breaking and entering. That was the first time I had ever done anything wrong in my life and it was a call for help.

In what way was it a call for help?

I'd just lost my family. I'd lost my job. I had nowhere to go. I wanted someone to talk to. I just *desperately* needed someone to talk to. I remember one night I was near a business premises. It was a full moon and I saw my reflection in the window. And I didn't like who I saw, so I picked up a railway sleeper that was lying there and tossed it through the window. It was *very* noisy. It probably hit point two on the Richter scale. Then I sat down and lit a cigarette and waited for someone to turn up, but no one came. I thought, 'I can't even get picked up properly!' So I went to the post office next door and rang the cops and told them that someone had broken into the premises next door. I went back into the building and sat down, lit another cigarette and just watched the action unfold. It was a circus. Security guards came, the police came, an ambulance. A policeman came in with a torch and put it on me, and said, 'Hey, come and have a look at this guy.'

You wanted to get caught.

Yes of course I did. I just wanted the whole thing to stop. I wanted the benders to stop. I wanted the noise in my head to stop. I wanted to get off the merry-go-round because it was going nowhere. I needed that break so bad . . .

Did you find someone to talk to?

I tried to talk to the judge but he wasn't interested. Within a short time of getting out of gaol I was in trouble again. I still wanted someone to talk to. I hoped that before I went completely mad someone might tell me what was happening. On one particular day I was drunk again and I went down to a Lotto place armed only with a bottle of whisky. I had all the staff line up against one wall and all the customers against another. I didn't know what I was doing and I really thought it was rather amusing that all these people were doing everything I was saying to them even though I didn't have a gun. Anyway the police came in, they assumed I was crazy and they took me to the psychiatric hospital. It was the first time I'd been to a mental hospital. I was in there a few more times . . . and then one time they put me in a different ward. It had a big high wall and razor wire and they put me on an anti-psychotic drug. The only way I can describe the effect is to say that everybody started to look as though they were characters from *Thunderbirds* . . . strange puppet-like movements. I was completely zapped for a number of weeks. Numb. Nothing. One guy eventually told me to put the medication under my tongue and then spit it out later. A little bit of sanity returned but because I was suddenly taking less medication, I started to have side effects. My arms and my head pulled back in strange spasm-like movements. My body was twisting in all directions as though it was trying to pull itself apart. I didn't know what was happening to me, so I went down to my bed. I tried to call out, but I couldn't because my jaw was also twisting sideways. Eventually a nurse came past and called the doctor straight away. He just pulled my pants down and stuck a needle straight into me. Then he called for my files and he realised that I was an alcoholic and shouldn't have been in that ward in the first place. I still believe that if he hadn't come along I'd still be walking around the halls of that hospital, believing that I was the person that they told me I was. Psychotic. Anti-social.

That was one scary time, but not just for me. It was scary to see human beings confined. It was scary to see them like sheep following one another. It was scary to see them so visibly changed by medication. It was scary to have doctors and psychiatrists with the power to say whether you could go or stay, whether you were better or worse. Society as a whole had no idea of what was going on behind those walls.

How did you eventually get out?

The probation officer came and saw me, and she

was in tears. She knew I was in the wrong ward and she was genuinely concerned for my welfare. She got me discharged and put into a hospital for drug and alcohol rehabilitation.

The real change in my life eventually came eight years ago. It was the turning point. The Holy Grail is something we all set out to achieve. Usually we set out on that quest when we are teenagers and we break away from home. Some of us go close to the Grail, some of actually see the Grail, some of us even touch the Grail, but most of us ride off on our horses dressed in armour and ride into the forest and don't come back for many years. Some never come back at all. But when you actually do come back, you're coming back with the wisdom of the world. And then you look around and you say, 'Oh, there's the Grail, it's been there the whole bloody time.' The question then is: 'What do you do with the Grail?'

When you know that answer, then you know who you are. The Holy Grail is knowing who you are. And I had my Grail the whole time.

How did you find out that you had it all the time?

At this time I was married to my current wife and my daughter was very young. We were renting a house and it was a lovely house. I was drinking so much that I couldn't work any more and so we were about to lose the house. Most of the furniture had already been taken away and put in storage. I was staying at the house and my wife was staying with her parents. I'd just been on a bender. Because I didn't eat properly when I was drinking, I often had ulcers – the drink ulcerates the stomach. One time when I was in hospital the doctor had counted 32 of them – peptic and duodenal ulcers. In any case, an ulcer had burst and I was feeling very ill. I was bleeding from the back passage and from the mouth as well. I felt like I was going to die and I felt like I *wanted* to die. My wife came over this particular day and said that I should get to hospital. I said I didn't want to go to hospital any more and that whatever happens, happens. My wife said she had decided to leave me if I didn't stop drinking.

I was feeling quite sorry for myself and I remember lying on a lounge that hadn't been packed up yet. And something flashed through my mind, 'Who's going to look after my wife and young daughter if I die?' Then I thought, 'Why the hell do you care, Patrick? Why all of a sudden start caring now? Your life's in disarray and you've lost another family.' I looked out the window and I saw my wife and daughter leaving, and the love that was inside me, that had been kept inside by the alcohol, poured out of me. And then I prayed. I said, 'If there's anyone up there, I know you've heard this many times before, but please just give me *one more chance.*' I was bleeding everywhere. I was trying hard not to fall asleep because I wasn't sure that I would ever wake up. I had always played with death up to that point, until there was nearly no return. This time I went so close I really could go no further and then I put my hand up and said, 'I've had enough.'

I don't know how I made it through the next day, but whatever happened to me at that point in time changed my life, because it came from *me*. It came from inside. No one else. It had to come from the soul . . . who I am as an individual. It was finding a strength inside that I never knew I had, and even today I am humbled by it. Very humbled by it . . . but it works. It wouldn't have worked if someone else had told me to give up drinking. That's the message I would like to get across to other people – if this son-of-a-bitch can do it then so can you. What I believe in has nothing to do with religion as it is today. It has something to do with the spiritual being that retains all the love. Pure love. That's all.

What was it like to be sober?

The first couple of years of not drinking was *the most painful period* because for the first time in my life I had to think. One of the torments of my past was my inability to think. When I was in the pub drinking, I could tell jokes and make people laugh, but when it came to anything important, I just put a humorous conclusion to it. The ceiling of the hotel was the limit of my thinking. I had dreadful headaches and people asked what was wrong. I had to say, 'You wouldn't believe it, but I'm trying to think.'

And *I didn't know anything*. I didn't know what it was like to be a human being in society any more. I also didn't know whether I had the courage to look after my wife and daughter. I didn't know whether I had the stamina. But I did know that I couldn't hold a drink in one hand and my family in the other.

Do you still suffer from manic depression?

Yes I do. I'm on lithium at the moment and on anti-depressant tablets. Sometimes when I get carried away, when I'm joking around with the family, I can feel that I can easily break through what I call the 'lithium barrier', but the lithium keeps it reasonably at bay, and my wife will notice when I am getting too high. My face gets red, my blood pressure starts to rise and I feel like a kettle on the boil . . . I can feel something happening in my system. It's not that I'd go and run around the streets with no clothes on, but the idea would be in my head.

232

I'm glad I've got someone who physically tells me, 'Patrick you're getting too high.' Then I might take more lithium, or I might find a quiet spot and relax to bring myself down. When the doctor put me on lithium she said, 'Patrick, from now on life is going to be very boring for you.'

You miss the highs . . .

I miss the energy and creativity of them. Nowadays instead of making something with my hands or whatever, I try to create reality as I know it. I try to create my life. I look at the reasons why I do the things that I do, I look at the way I meet people and talk with them, I look at the directions I want to go in and the ones that I don't. I don't believe that you have to look at everything in your life, but I do believe that from going through what I have, I now know my dark side.

What has knowing that dark side brought to your life?

Many things. A bit more confidence in knowing my boundaries. And also depth. When I have ordinary everyday conversations with people, like my neighbours, I am aware that sometimes I have to pull back the reins because I want more out of the conversation. Everyday conversations are boring. I see the darkness as a depth and I long for that depth in all my interactions. I find I have a craving for it. The physical plane doesn't do it for me. Call it spirituality or whatever, but there is something that I saw as a homeless alcoholic . . . a serenity . . . not fighting any more who you are, but giving in. To hell with what people think of you.

So you don't find that depth and serenity in everyday interactions between people?

No. My soul needs education. My soul needs growth. My soul needs food. I don't know what that food is.

Perhaps it is knowledge. Perhaps it is when you meet with other people and you know that person has been through similar experiences and you can sense a deep connection with them. The darkness is my food – it is the unknown place that we are all frightened to go to. I often wonder why I got this far and others didn't. What is it about Patrick that made me survive this distance?

What do you think it is?

I think it has something to do with my destiny. Perhaps it was simply the destiny of others to die. They fulfilled their role and it was time for them to move on. I don't think I've quite fulfilled my destiny yet. I've learnt from so many wonderful experiences, but I've got to put it to some use. What can I do with it? I've tried to get into the next place in this universe but they wouldn't let me in. I took an overdose once. I had my stomach pumped and a psychiatrist came to see me and he said, 'Young man, you are so lucky to be alive, we got you in just the nick of time. God must have held you in the palm of his hand.' I replied, 'Well if he is, he's bloody crushing me!' That's how it felt.

So you feel there is something still left for you to complete?

Yes. And it could be just to start something . . . that would be enough. I don't know. I believe I have a very strong future ahead of me. I believe I am very fortunate in that sense – the pain of my experiences has given me a lot of wisdom and I hope that one day I can pass some of that on to people who have not yet seen the light at the end of tunnel.

I feel very fortunate and I feel excited about the future.

David

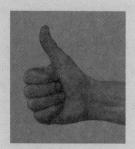

David is 50 years old and has been diagnosed with schizophrenia. He hopes that in being interviewed he might help others to see that regardless of how desperate their circumstances, there is always a hope that life may turn around. In his work and in his life David now gives to others. *'This photo of the "thumbs up" is for hope and for my son. I carry a photo of him as a little boy in my wallet. In it he is proudly giving me the thumbs up.'*

I fear the wrath of man but much more I fear the wrath of God.

If there is a hell I was heading there.

This is the beginning of my story . . .

When I was thirteen years old I lived happily with my family. I was in the rowing club at high school and also the army cadets. I wasn't a very good soldier because I didn't like orders being yelled at me, but all the same I thought I looked pretty spiffy in my uniform and my shiny black boots. Sometimes when I caught the bus home from school I was still wearing my cadet uniform and a young lady by the name of Barbara would glance at me. She had red hair. She was about my age and we became very friendly. She was a great girl, but I wasn't very experienced with girls and so I never got around to asking her home for dinner.

Later on Barbara will become significant in this story.

When I was fourteen my life turned upside down. Dad got a job in Brisbane and I moved there with my eldest sister and father while Mum and the rest of the family stayed at home. Suddenly I was in a new city, in a new suburb and in a rented house. My father and sister were both working long hours and I remember coming home from school to an empty house. I felt very isolated, lonely and abandoned. And there was no Barbara there either.

I went to a high school where they wanted me to do French. I hadn't done a language so I was a year behind, which I didn't like. Then I went to another high school and I was able to enrol without doing a language. I settled in and made some great friends.

But then Mum and the rest of the family joined us, so we had to move to a new house and I had to change schools *again*. In biology class I met a girl and she introduced herself as Barbara. She had blonde hair. She showed me her right arm, which had been badly scarred by a burn. I remember thinking how much it must have hurt her. I wanted to ask her out but I didn't. In another class I smiled at a boy in the back row because he was clowning around but rather than smile back, he took an instant dislike to me. He had a gang of mates and they always had it in for me. I was thin and frail then and I was scared of him. As a result I started to abscond from school with some mates and I began drinking heavily. We were pisspots. At the end of that year I passed only two subjects. It was very detrimental to my education.

I left school and became a junior store person for a while, but I knew I really wanted a trade. I'd always been interested in photography, so I got an apprenticeship in photography. I finished that and then started my working life. With the extra money, I could party and drink more. On Friday nights we regularly went to dances and on one occasion a mate and I met two girls. He paired up with one of them and I paired up with the other. She had jet-black hair. I fell in love with her on the spot. She was a lovely girl and I remember kissing her, but she wouldn't speak to me. I asked her name but for some reason she wouldn't tell me. Then within half an hour the two girls had to leave. I remember calling out to her as she was leaving, 'I love you! I love you!' I saw her again later outside the hall and I asked 'Can I see you? Can I have your phone number?' But she wouldn't speak and I still don't know her name.

I was getting older and more experienced at talking to girls. At one dance I saw one of my mates dancing with a girl and kissing her. She was quite a pretty girl. Later on I saw her standing on her own and I thought, 'Well what's good for my mate is good for me!' I went up to her and asked her to dance. We gradually got to know each other better. Her name was Diane and we came to love each other. When her parents decided to move to Sydney, she didn't want to go with them because of her relationship with me, and so we moved in together at quite a young age.

We lived together for a number of years. I worked hard at my job and even got another part-time job. I bought a speedboat and we often went water skiing. Diane even learnt to drive the boat. Life was great and after a time we got married. At first we lived in a small flat and went without lots of things to save for a house. I got a good job with the government, sold the speedboat and put a deposit on some land.

While we were living in the flat, saving hard, we knew a woman in the house across the road. We were friendly but not too friendly. At one time she came to me and said, 'The girl who's living with us is unwell, could you look in on her while we're away and see that she's alright.' I thought it was strange that she was asking me for help with this girl, so I told her that I'd have to ask my wife, as I wasn't sure that she would approve of it. Nothing came of it, but I remember my wife being a little concerned about the situation.

I also joined the lifesavers and was with them for about six years. I enjoyed rowing a surfboat in the carnivals on Sundays. I was a little upset that my wife wouldn't mix in with the lifesaving people though. I was making nice friends and I would have liked it if she'd joined in too, but she was the sort of person who preferred to stay home and read.

We moved to the new house. Not long after, I quit lifesaving and we started doing up the house. We put the fences up and established the garden. It was a lovely house. Everything in our lives was going as planned. I was earning good money and it seemed like the right time to have a child. Diane got pregnant and we fixed up a nursery in the house.

When the time came for the birth of the child I was in the delivery room. I saw the baby being born and it was a little girl. But I could see straight away that the doctor was very upset. The baby had birth defects and wasn't well. She had some sort of syndrome that meant she would be retarded. The next eighteen days were pure hell, travelling back and forth to the hospital in the city. After seventeen days they let us move her to a hospital closer to home. And on the eighteenth day the baby died. When the baby was dying we were put in a special room. She died a very long slow painful death in my wife's arms. It was *so* drawn out. I remember the little baby gasping for air. There were times I thought it would be so much more humane if I could just put my hand over her mouth and make it quick for her. It just took so long for the little girl to die. Afterwards I remember the doctor showing us books of photos with people who had the same syndrome. He said, 'This is what she would have looked like. She's done you a favour by dying. You're lucky she has passed away because otherwise you would have had a severely handi-capped child on your hands.' A priest was with us at the time, and I would have liked him to say a prayer or something, but he didn't say a thing. I'm sure the priest probably did bless her and put her before God. I'm sure she's in heaven now.

After the death of the baby, things changed between Diane and me. She was never the same again. I think she actually hated me or blamed me for the baby's prob-lems. But we stayed together. I remember one day driving home from work and realising that my wife was in *deep* trouble. I felt the only way I had of helping her was to give her another baby. So I started eating Mars Bars (for energy) on the way home from work and trying really hard to have lots of sex and get her pregnant again. She did get pregnant again but after about four months she miscarried. She was back at the same hospital where she had lost the first baby.

When Diane got home this time the situation was just terrible. She was emotionally distraught, hurt and depressed. We kept trying for another baby even though sex was now a dreadful chore and damaging to our relationship. Nothing about it was fun. However, she did get pregnant again.

When she was well into the pregnancy with our third child I knew I had to follow my dream of becoming a famous photographer. I felt that once the child was born I would no longer have the opportunity to do so. So I chucked in a damn good job, started studying photography at college and working as a freelance pho-tographer. Although I was technically brilliant in the darkroom I have to admit that my photographs were really pretty average. They never turned out like I had imagined them. My career was consequently very short-lived and we had to sell our beautiful house. We no longer had a home and it seemed everything we had planned for in our lives had gone wrong.

We moved in with my grandmother but that didn't work out either and so we ended up in a rented caravan in a caravan park. Things were pretty grim. I don't know what went wrong with me around this time, but I just wasn't 'with it' any more. I think this was the beginning of my mental illness. My life was falling apart. I was unemployed. Thank goodness for Diane though, because she got us a house from the Department of Housing just before the baby was born. It was a dump in comparison to the house we had, but it was still a fine place.

I'm not sure of the time frame here, but I remember that before the birth of the first baby I had been seeing a psychiatrist occasionally. He had thought it might be good to talk with me about our family. He diagnosed me with manic depression and he put me on medication even though I remember feeling perfectly all right then. But as things had progressed in my life I *did* become very depressed. My wife hated me, two babies had died, we'd lost the house, and I was unemployed. I became a regular patient of the psychiatrist.

Our third child was born and it was a lovely little boy and he was perfect. Fourteen months later we had a little girl and she was perfect too. But our marriage wasn't good. We were strangers. I was beginning to lose it. I had started telling Diane that I thought I was going to have two wives. It was understandable that she was increasingly angry and nasty and wouldn't talk to me any more. She wanted to be *the* one and definitely not part of a harem! In any case, I got a job again, and even though it was a struggle, we built another house.

Then one night I came home from work. Diane had called the police in the hope that they would be able to throw me out. She wanted the house and the kids but she didn't want me there any more. But when the police said that throwing me out was not within their jurisdiction, she took the kids and left. As a result I became very ill and almost immediately ended up in the psychiatric hospital. I had started acting irrationally. I took my clothes off and ran around the streets naked. One time I caught a train to see my doctor and I took my clothes off in the train. I thought I *had* to do these things. This may have been the real beginning of my mental illness but I still think it started at the death of my first child. It had been such a traumatic event in my life and I had no way of coping with it.

After I came out of hospital, I stayed with my parents. In the interim Diane had moved back into the house and had slapped a restraining order on me. It was devastating. Having all that trouble in the beginning and then having two beautiful little children . . . and then not seeing them . . .

. . . and this is where it gets really bad . . . hence my quote at the beginning . . .

I started thinking I was wired and that a lady was watching me electronically and hearing everything I did. She was watching via a sort of satellite. I had some kind of implant in me so that she could watch what I was doing and hear what I was saying. She was monitoring me. I don't know where these ideas came from, whether from songs on the radio or . . . there was a song by The Police that really affected me . . . about someone watching me . . .

Anyway, I started acting things out because I had to help this woman. She was exceptionally wealthy and I believed that by doing the things that she wanted me to do, I would meet her and have a life of wealth, fame and power.

At one time I went to a party that was held by an organisation of which I was a member. I had some nice friends there, all of whom had similar marital problems. I had a few drinks and I thought I had to do something in order to help this lady who was watching me. Circumstances just seemed to fall into place at the time and I knew I *had* to do it. I had no choice. Consequently I committed a crime at the party and was caught. I remember one of the people there spitting in my face and I knew that I deserved it. Why did I do that? Why did I do that? I knew it was wrong but I couldn't stop it.

I went home to my parents' place afterwards and the next moment the police were at the door. I was taken to the police station and charged, but because I had no previous convictions the judge put me on probation.

I got through my probation period and then started going to a religious organisation. At their regular Sunday meetings I started to get messages from the woman who was watching me. She told me that I would be able to meet with her if I could go to gaol. I had to break the law and go to gaol to meet this lady. How insane is that? . . . but I didn't see it as insane at the time. I won't go into the details . . . but I was convicted of three offences all on the one day. I knew it was all dreadfully wrong but I thought I *had* to do it.

Naturally enough I was on my way to gaol – a prison house for the criminally insane. I got five years. And I didn't meet the woman there. During that time I saw a psychiatrist and he diagnosed me with schizophrenia. We talked about everything that had happened and I was put on anti-psychotic and other medication. But the medication didn't really have any effect on my thoughts. Even to this day my thoughts are associated with the lady who watches me.

At the age of 41, after eighteen months of my sentence, I got out of gaol and spent the remaining time on parole. My life had deteriorated so much from what I had been and my family was very disappointed in me. I had wanted to be a family man. I had been a lifesaver. I had been an asset to the community. I detested myself for what I had done.

All this time I'd had my name down for a Department of Housing flat and when I got out of prison it finally came through. And so I started a life on my own, seeing a psychiatrist and a parole officer. I also did an offenders rehabilitation course. It was full-on stuff and I had to talk about what I had done. It made me realise that I'd gone so low – that I'd hit rock bottom.

For the next seven years or so of my life I sulked in my flat. Every day was much the same. I'd sleep in till about eleven o'clock, get up and have a coffee and a bit of lunch, watch some television, and then go back to bed. That was about it. I was very lonely and isolated and felt very hurt. I wasn't very proud of myself. My self-esteem was very low. I only went out if I had an appointment with my psychiatrist. I took my medication and just existed.

In my mind though, I milled endlessly over the past. I had the notion that all these Barbaras – the Barbara on the bus, the Barbara in the biology class, the girl at the dance with jet-black hair and the girl across the road from the flat – were all the same girl. I was quite sure that I'd figured out that this special lady who was watching me was actually the same Barbara I had met all those times throughout the years – except with different hair colour. My doctor assured me that this was not the case and that the Barbara who was watching me was actually a delusion. He also told me that these four girls were all *different* girls.

After years of talking with my doctor about it and his assurance that the lady was a delusion, I've now come to the conclusion that maybe it isn't Barbara after all, and that maybe there is no one watching me. I was trying to act out all these things to help her but I really just don't know any more. I tried my best to help her and that's all I can do. I kept going from one special event to another thinking that one day I would meet her, but I never have, and quite frankly I don't have the energy to work it all out any more. I thought I was clever and knew all the answers but I no longer think I do.

Another part of my mental illness – it just came into my head from nowhere – was the thought that I was going to be on a manned mission to Mars. My doctor calls it a 'delusion of grandeur'. I was sure I was going to be someone pretty important – I thought I would be taken to England to study and then be taken on to America to become an astronaut. But over that seven-year period of sulking, I have gradually aged and I am beginning to realise that I've probably missed my opportunity to go to Mars. I'm 50 now, and I assume that by the time I'm 55, I'll definitely be too old. The delusion is taking care of itself as I mature! But it was nice to think that I could have gone to Mars. It would have been a nice adventure. I've read lots of books on Mars at the library and have been very interested to research the Mars probes on the Internet. One day I am sure they *will* do a manned mission to Mars, but I don't think I will be on it. There is a movie with Clint Eastwood in it called *Space Cowboys*. It is about these geriatric guys who go on a space mission – that gave me hope for a moment . . . but I'm slowly realising that I'm not going to be all that important after all. I'm just an ordinary bloke like everybody else.

And then after seven years of sulking in my flat came September 11 2001 . . .

It really rocked my boat. It affected me deeply. I was watching television and it started coming through live from New York and I was so horrified at the scale of the event and the sheer number of victims. Innocent people going to work. It shocked me so much that the world had become such a dangerous place. It knocked me off my fence . . .

After that event I went to church with one of my neighbours and have been going ever since. Who was there to turn to after such horror but the Lord? The message is that if we genuinely seek the Lord and try to live by his ways we'll be forgiven for our sins. And that is the best thing that has been offered to me to date. Forgiveness, for me, is redemption from sin. I have repented for my past and I am 'born again'. I imagine there are people who would definitely never forgive me for what I have done, but God *does* offer forgiveness and gives me a new beginning. I can start a new life.

I regularly go to church and seek the Lord's direction in my life. I have some nice friends in the church and they know I have a mental illness and take medication. They don't know the nature of it, but they're still very supportive and understanding. I'm being invited to barbecues and social functions.

I still live alone but I don't feel lonely any more.

I know some people probably wouldn't understand this, but I feel the Lord's comfort. I didn't have that feeling of comfort before, but I do now. And I also have hope. I had always thought that with all the things I had done and with events in the world like September 11, that there was no hope. But now there is hope . . . hope that I won't be damned to hell. Some people find it in meditation, some people find it in other things . . . I don't know, but I've found *my* spot and I even believe that when the Lord is ready he will find me a nice lady. My focus now is on pleasing the Lord.

I changed my medication around the same time as September 11, but my psychiatrist doesn't think the medication could have such a profound effect. The only other thing that I can put it down to is the Lord.

I still see myself as someone living with schizophrenia. I take my medication and I see my doctor one week and my caseworker the next. I tell them every little thing I'm thinking about. I don't hold back. I think it's important to lay it all on the line so they can say, 'Hey David, you're going off on a tangent.'

Perhaps this is delusional as well, but sometimes people are rude to me. I was brought up to be friendly and polite, but I've had a lot of people, including Christians, who are damn rude and arrogant to me. I wonder whether they are preparing me for an ordeal I might have to go through or are trying to help me in some way. Perhaps I have to fight World War Three all on my own overseas. I don't know. But I never repay rudeness with rudeness. Our Saviour says you should love your enemies. I always try to stay friendly and show love to all people.

Things are going really well in my life now. I'm working again. I got a nice tax return cheque this year and I was able to buy a clarinet. I've got a beginner's book and I'm teaching myself how to play. I also hope to have lessons one day. I've also acquired an old hymn book and I'm learning to play the melodies . . . and I'm driving my neighbours crazy at the same time! One of my favourites is *How Great Thou Art*. It is a hymn based on an old Swedish folk melody. My grandmother used to sing it to me when I was a little boy. I played it at my father's birthday a couple of months ago.

Coralie

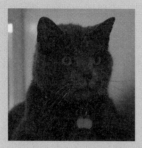

Coralie is 57 years old. She has had a very turbulent and yet exciting life. She has travelled extensively through Europe, the US, UK and Asia. She feels privileged to have had three children and a wonderful husband. She has two grandchildren. *'I love all cats. Max, my oldest cat, is thirteen years old now. He is very important to me. He was given to me so that I wouldn't feel lonely when my husband passed away. At the moment I have seven cats, because I've also taken in a stray who presented me with five kittens.'*

Some important things

Some important things happened when I was seventeen. I was in my final year at school and I fell in love and got married. My husband was my soul mate and I loved him dearly. His job took him interstate and I went with him. I wanted to be a pharmacist, so I went to university and completed a science degree. However, when I finished studying, my biological clock was going beserk. I wanted very much to have children and so that's what we decided to do. We had three children in just over two years.

Our first-born was Tania, our second-born was Peter and our third-born was Kylie. Kylie died from heart failure when she was four years old and Peter was diagnosed with leukaemia when he was two and a half. After a really long battle he lost his fight for life just before his eighth birthday. Tania has gone on to produce two wonderful grandchildren.

But it was the death of my husband in '93 that really

got to me. I suppose that's where the depression really began, although I believe it may actually have started after my daughter died. At that time the doctor had simply said to me, 'Go home. Get on with life. Take care of your family.' I was probably depressed from that point but didn't really acknowledge it.

What was it that had changed after your daughter's death.

My thoughts were very different.

In what way?

I constantly thought of suicide. I often thought of suiciding with Peter, particularly when things with him weren't getting any better. He had an awful lot of pain, and getting drugs to alleviate that pain was a difficult process. And we also had to inject him with morphine at home. It put a lot of a pressure on me. I thought suicide wasn't necessarily an easier way out . . . it was just a better way out . . . for Peter.

But it was when my husband died two days before Christmas in '93, that I just completely lost it. I fell into a black hole. My GP sent a psychiatrist to see me and he had me detained. He felt I was unsafe to myself and to others and that was definitely a reason for detaining me. He called an ambulance to take me to hospital.

Were you detained immediately after your husband's death?

Straight after the funeral. But when the ambulance arrived, they wouldn't take me to hospital because I was a detained person.

Why?

I guess it was that detained people are uncontrollable.

Were you uncontrollable?

Oh no! I was almost catatonic . . . and so I had to go to hospital in a police car. But the really ridiculous thing about that was that I'd just had major surgery from a car accident and I was in a plaster cast from my hip to my ankle. They had great trouble getting me into the back of the police car and the officer who got in the back with me had to nurse my leg. The police knew how stupid the whole thing was, because I could hardly move! Six weeks later, when the psychiatrist who had detained me found out what had happened, he wrote a scathing letter to the ambulance people and we got a formal apology.

Anyway, I was so embarrassed because I'd never been in trouble with the police before, so when we got to the hospital the police officer said, 'Just hang on to my arm and we'll walk through emergency here and they'll just think we're friends. Nobody will know that you're in trouble.' And that's exactly what we did. And that helped. The police were excellent.

What happened once you were in hospital?

While I was in hospital I was put on antidepressants and given counselling, but it didn't really shift my mood at all. I was still very suicidal. When I got home there was no follow-up other than my private psychiatrist. My mood escalated and it was really only a matter of months before I was in again.

Should there have been some follow-up?

There should have been follow-up but they didn't do it in those days. They didn't have the resources or perhaps they hadn't even thought of it. That's only twelve years ago . . . but they do it now.

I used to spend eight weeks in hospital after a suicide attempt, get out, then back to hospital . . . and this pattern went on year after year. When I was at home I basically just sat in the dark. I didn't open the curtains. I didn't answer the phone or anything. I did nothing.

How did you survive in terms of basic essentials such as food?

I had one friend who I'd met when I was in hospital the first time. She's still a very close friend today. She and her husband basically took me on board. They always made sure there was enough food in the house . . . though I didn't really eat . . . I lost an awful lot of weight during that time.

There were also times when my girlfriend recognised that there was something wrong with me. At one stage she apparently rang me and I guess I must have sounded different or irrational. She said to her husband that they had to come over. And they came over. I must have been at the front door and they said that they wanted to come in, but I didn't know how to open the door . . . they had to stand there for a long time before I understood how to use the key to open the door.

Had you taken something?

No. That was my operating mode. Apparently they took me home to their place and fed me soup, but I have no recollection of this. Apparently I did not even know what utensils were for. They took me to my GP. I was still basically comatose, and the GP got an ambulance and I was taken to hospital. I had no drugs in my blood; it was just some sort of catatonic state. I have them occasionally.

She also decided to drag me out of the house and into a swimming pool. I stood in the shallow end for six months. Just standing. And she'd sit there with me. That's just what she did. And she persevered with me, which I thought was fantastic. I guess she was the only one who could communicate with me at the level I was on.

. . . even if that communication was simply to sit with you.

Yeah. My daughter wasn't able to cope with me. She was just a wreck. When I saw my grandchildren I indicated that I wanted to kill them too. In my state of mind at the time I thought that it was quite reasonable to kill them so that they wouldn't have the pain of this world.

The pain of this world
What *was* the pain of this world that you wished to protect them from?

My husband had HIV and he died from AIDS. And he had it because he was a haemophiliac . . . and he had it because I had given him the transfusion at home. My daughter's son is also a haemophiliac and when I was really ill, I thought it would be a good idea if he didn't live any longer. My daughter quite naturally lost all faith in me . . . her reaction was understandable. I'm not critical of her at all.

Did the fact that you had given your husband the transfusion that had carried the HIV virus contribute to your pain?

Yes, very much so. I still accuse myself of doing it to him. I still feel guilty. I haven't been able to forgive myself yet.

Did your husband blame you?

Oh no. Heavens no! He blamed the people who were responsible . . . the Red Cross . . . CSL[17] . . . I think in '84 they didn't yet have a name for AIDS, but they knew that something was in their blood stocks that definitely wasn't good and shouldn't be in there. They'd given us the contaminated stuff to have at home and only afterwards recalled it all.

In '84 my husband had to go in to have a blood test

---

17 Commonwealth Serum Laboratories

and they said, 'If we don't call you, you'll know that you don't have any problems, and if we do, well we'll take it from there.' We didn't hear anything and so we assumed everything was fine. But then in '86, out of the blue, we got a phone call saying, 'Oh we forgot to tell you that your blood is HIV positive.' Of course we'd been practising unsafe sex during that time because we were a monogamous couple and I'd had a hysterectomy. So I was in trouble too.

And then eventually we found out that he also had Hepatitis A, Hepatitis B and Hepatitis C. No one had told us. And it wasn't that I was so concerned for myself. What about our daughter? What if we had given our daughter AIDS or Hep B or C? We didn't keep the cutlery separate or anything like that. But fortunately nothing happened.

We had a lot of anger towards CSL and the Red Cross ... they were ultimately taken to court by the Haemophilia Association of Australia on behalf of all the haemophiliacs who got AIDS ... and they lost. Everyone got a payout.

Did that payout come before your husband's death?

Only just. It helped to pay for all things we tried in order to save him.

How did the period from your husband's diagnosis to his death affect *you*?

It was shocking. I had to seek help. The Haemophilia Association had a psychiatrist and I managed to tap in to him. He was really good. He kept me alive. We talked about all the things that were bothering me and he encouraged me to keep going. He did put me in hospital a couple of times for a bit of a rest. I saw him every week because the tension at home was so bad. I probably wouldn't have got through that period without him, because I was constantly suicidal. I wouldn't have done anything then, but it was always in my mind. Constantly. It was just like a record that went over and over and over and never ended: 'Kill yourself. Kill yourself. Kill yourself.'

Why do you think that was?

Sometimes I wonder if it was an easy way out.

Had those thoughts stayed with you since the death of your children?

No. They had definitely lifted. I had been involved with my daughter's life and I had just continued on. And looking after a haemophiliac was quite a constant chore too.

What was that like?

You have to give transfusions of Factor 8. It's Factor 8 that's missing. I had to put it in like a natural transfusion as many times as my husband was having a bleed or thought he was having a bleed. My husband's bleeds were mostly internal – a joint would blow out for instance.

Did that come from a bump or injury?

No, it didn't have to be anything. I would do transfusions at two in the morning, at five in the morning . . . whatever. He was always on my mind, 'Do I have to do it again today?' If I stopped the bleed with one dose, I knew that I would probably have to do three or four follow-ups. One bottle only has a half-life of twelve hours, so I had to give a real cover to stop the bleed altogether. And then there was traipsing into the hospital to get more stuff . . . seeing the doctor . . .

Did you have to be qualified to transfuse?

I learnt how to do it. They gave me an orange to practise on . . . which I can tell you is *nothing* like a vein! There is *no* resemblance between an orange and a vein! They were very turbulent times but we didn't let them rule our lives. We just got on with it. My husband had a job . . . we worked around that . . . we travelled . . . I even transfused him on long flights to England.

But it is interesting that my daughter believed that it wouldn't be any bother to her if she *did* have a son with haemophilia . . . and I was so sad that I had passed that impression on to her, because it *is* a demanding job. She's only just discovering that now.

But things changed after your husband was diagnosed with HIV.

Yes. He haemorrhaged all the time. That's an enormous thing. He had haemorrhaged all his life but with the HIV it got worse. He had mood swings because he was depressed but he wouldn't take anything for it. He was losing a lot of weight and just generally didn't seem able to help himself or let anyone else help him, other than me.

And he wouldn't talk about what was going on at all. It was the 'Grim Reaper' time and the stigma of AIDS was so severe that we just couldn't mention it. Having to watch those commercials on TV was just horrible, particularly for my husband. I think they made him feel like a non-person. The only people who knew that he had AIDS were our really close family members. We didn't have anyone to share with. My daughter and I were under immense pressure on a daily basis.

I was also aware that he would have a reduced life expectancy, but I don't think *he* was. He thought he was going to live for a long time . . . At first I thought he should accept that he was going to die, but then I thought, 'Well if he's coping this way, let him cope this way.'

And then gradually during the five years or so before his death, the AIDS started to affect his brain. He started to really lose it. He spent money for no reason. He lost all logic. He did strange things. I think it was a form of dementia because a couple of times I woke up in the middle of the night and he was trying to suffocate me with a pillow. I ended up having to get Enduring Power of Attorney. He had been the funniest and happiest human being you could ever meet and people absolutely adored him. The day we buried him there were over 1000 people at the church . . . out on the road . . . everywhere . . .

Black dog
Although you feel that your depression began with your husband's death, before then there had been a tremendous . . .

. . . pressure . . .

. . . would you have thought of yourself as someone living with mental illness during that period?

I guess if you'd asked my psychiatrist he would probably have put a label on me as being severely depressed, but I didn't see myself in that way. Certainly not then. Because I still had to exist: work, shop, iron, keep the family together. I didn't see myself as having anything really wrong with me prior to his death, other than an enormous amount of stress in my life. It wasn't until after his death when my depression wouldn't subside and I had mood swings that went from manic activity into very low depression that I realised something was really wrong. My brain felt as though it was scrambled and I couldn't think logically. I was labelled as bipolar.

Do you see a connection between your experiences and the onset of bipolar?

I do see a connection. A *big* connection now. It's actually not uncommon for depression to turn into bipolar when you've suffered a lot of trauma. But I've only found that out as I've been working more and more in the mental health arena. Trauma is definitely going to affect a person, and the more you have, the more severely you will be affected.

Depression I feel is a complete and utter overload. It is what people used to call a 'nervous breakdown'. A lot of the old people still refer to it as a nervous breakdown. I think those words have the sense that you're breaking down for a reason. But if you're depressed, people tend to think, 'Well so what . . . you're *just* depressed!' The word 'depression' makes light of what it actually is. Depression is *so* many things: it's the way you feel, it's that terrible dragging agonising emotional pain that you're in, it's the black hole . . .

What name would *you* give it?

What did Churchill call it? . . . Black Dog! It needs a more catastrophic word, because that in turn would have people thinking more about mental illness.

Earlier in the interview you spoke of a pattern of attempted suicide and then hospitalisation.

The last time I nearly killed myself was eighteen months ago. I gassed myself in the car. I spent a very long time in intensive care at the time and killed off some brain cells. I was sick for a long time. I don't remember much about it actually, I just know that I did it.

Suicide has always been a quick thing for me. I think and then I do. About everything else I am pretty slow and casual, but suicide is different. If I say, 'I want to go now,' then I have to go now.

In my mind, the only way I can justify the death of my children is that for them, wherever they may be, time does not exist. I imagine that when I die they will recognise me as the person they last saw two minutes ago. I believe that dying and being with them again, is a better thing than living. I see it as a form of euthanasia. I always want to go and be with my husband and the kids. I have not been able to stop that. It becomes a demanding thought. It didn't make sense for kids to die. Kids don't die before their parents . . . it's not supposed to happen . . . but I know it does . . .

. . . but it's been eighteen months since my last suicide attempt. It's been the longest time that I've been out of hospital. That's a positive thing because hospitalisation has always felt very dehumanising.

Dehumanisation

I have always been detained, and that means I have always been an *involuntary* patient. It means you can't change your mind. You can't say 'no'. And you can't go anywhere. You have no privileges. You have an escort wherever you go. If you don't take your medication you are given an injection. You're strip-searched. Sometimes body cavities are searched. They take away all your belts, bras, shoelaces . . . anything you can tie up and use as a weapon against yourself.

The first time I was detained with my leg in a cast, I complained that it was very painful. They said that it was in my mind because I was grieving. But when I got discharged and went to see my orthopaedic surgeon, I found out it was actually broken again and I had to have it reset. There was a total disregard of anything I said. I know of people who have not been believed, who have then taken overdoses and died.

Another lockup ward I've been on was horrendous. You don't have any clothes. They'll only bring them to you if they see fit. You wear whatever they give you. The bedroom is locked and you only have cold showers with a nurse in there watching you. That still happens.

Another particular time I remember as clear as day. I was on a mixed ward . . . it was summer and they took my bra away and my T-shirt showed my boobs . . . they took my belt and my trousers kept falling down . . . they had no doors on the showers and toilets . . . a male could have walked in any time he felt like it.

My friend brought up some clothing for me and with it she brought my son's little teddy bear. I am not sure why she did that, but she did it anyway. A nurse who was working out what items I could have in my little space, got the teddy bear and drop-kicked it across the room. He waited to see what I would do.

Was he taunting you?

Yeah. He was bad. He wanted a reaction from me. He knew the teddy bear was special.

. . . and the other thing he did to me. My brother came to see me and I didn't know the rules. The nurse pointed to a spot on the floor and said, 'Stand there!' The spot was some distance from a door that allowed my brother to come in. I thought that I was standing exactly where he told me, but he kept telling me that it wasn't the right spot. I kept changing where I was standing but I just couldn't please him. Eventually he sent me back into the ward and decided he wouldn't let my brother come in to visit me. I was really distressed because I thought I wasn't going to see him. Next thing, for reasons I am not quite sure of, I was ushered back out to see my brother. My brother is a big guy and he was really angry. Perhaps my brother had persuaded him, but I don't know.

How did his treatment affect you at a time when you were already suffering?

It made me angry. And even sicker. At that time I just withdrew even further. I curled up in a little ball, because I wasn't going to let him hurt me. I wasn't going to let him make me stay there any longer than I had to. Sometimes I actually came out of hospital sicker than when I went in because such incidents left me feeling even more worthless. Even just being on a psychiatric ward was really traumatising for me particularly when I'd never been there before.

Was the attitude of this nurse common in the treatment of detained patients?

This nurse wasn't the rule, but there *are* a number of them. But there are also better ones.

How are they different?

They'd encourage you to get better. They gave you hope that you would get well again and get out of there. They would generally make it easier for you. If they had to be in the shower with you, they might turn their back and chat with you so that it wasn't an embarrassing thing. They took their time with you, they never harassed you, they might take you for a walk. That sort of thing had a big impact for your recovery. They made you feel that it was important that you got well. The nasty ones couldn't have cared less whether you got well or not. They hated you.

Did these experiences leave you with any general thoughts about the nature of psychiatric care?

I think care providers must be mindful of the ways that their practices and policies might bring about re-traumatisation. I don't think they realise that symptoms and negative behaviour are *already* an adaptation to traumatic events. Negative behaviour should therefore be viewed as a strength rather than as a fault.

A lot of people come into psychiatric wards and

act out violently for example. These people get a very bad reputation with the nurses on the ward. The nurses don't have a lot of time for them. Service providers have to remember that acting out is part of the symptoms. People are trying to manage the experience of trauma when they're acting out, they're trying to communicate and once you break through that they'll stop acting out. Service providers must help people to create safe spaces in which they can manage their symptoms.

Being treated well is also the realisation that you need following up when you leave hospital . . . you may be linked with a key worker who sees you weekly and supports you . . . I didn't have anything like that when I came out the first time and that was a major problem for me. And that would have been the same for anyone else during that era. But there's certainly been a big improvement in our system since then. We now have a system that allows people who are still pretty unwell to be back in the community, but with nurses who come out every day to look after them. That can go on for a number of weeks after a hospitalisation. But key workers work well for me.

In what way?

They are very accessible. They are someone I can ring when I am sliding and they can help to pick me up. They can remind you of all the things you can do to help yourself – have a drink with a friend, walk on the beach, listen to music. But generally when people contact their key worker, they've tried all that stuff, and are looking for extra help to get over the hurdle. Having that contact is very supportive. Key workers might even come out to the house. In my opinion there aren't enough of them!

But I don't have a key worker now. I just have my psychiatrist and my GP. I didn't necessarily get discharged from my key worker, but rather I got passed on to a GP who is able to do mental health . . . that works very well for me. My psychiatrist talks to the GP and the GP talks back to the psychiatrist. The GP also talks to the chemist so that I get my medication . . . because I'm not allowed to have my medication for longer than a week at a time . . . that's part of the stigma . . . I often used to accumulate drugs for attempting suicide . . . so I am only allowed to collect my medication every week now. It's a bit of a pain.

I'd just like to make the point that as far as dealing with service providers goes, I think consumers need to recognise that their mental illness, particularly if they have depression, makes it difficult for them to be assertive. When they go to the doctor they'll probably do whatever they're told to do, even if inside they're thinking, 'I don't want to do that.' They need to be able to learn to be assertive. They can do this by taking classes for instance.

Are you assertive with your care providers?

Oh yeah. A lot more than I ever was. If I don't want to do something now, I say, 'No, I don't want to do that.' Then they'll try all sorts of things to get you to say yes or come up with a different idea.

What if they continue to insist on it?

I'd still say no. But I suppose if they feel I'm *really* wrong, I'd probably be detained.

Do you see that as a major drawback to being assertive?

Always . . . and that does happen to people . . . many times. And it's happened to me. It's called 'not having insight'. You have to be careful not to assert yourself in an angry way. If you do it in a fairly placid, controlled and yet strong voice and add your reasons as to why you feel that way, they *will* listen

Have you ever said 'no' to medication?

Yes.

What was the outcome?

I was detained. Again, they felt that I didn't have enough insight.

Did *you* feel that you had enough insight?

Yeah. I did.

Why did you say no to that particular medication?

I'd done research on the Internet and I didn't like the list of side effects. Their response was that I had to endure the side effects because this drug was good for me.

Did you feel that being detained was warranted?

I think it was a bit over the top. But then again I suppose I have to take the professionals' judgement in mind, because there were times I could have been wrong. Quite often people can think that they're doing really well when they're not.

I can remember one time I was at a fairly high-powered meeting, and when the meeting ended, the chair of the meeting said to me, 'I'd like a chat, Coralie.' So we went down to her office and had a chat and she said, 'Well I'm sorry but I've got to detain you.' As far as she was concerned my behaviour had altered. I didn't feel it was justified at that time. I wasn't talking about suicide or anything. I spent six weeks in hospital.

She detained you there and then?

Yes they have to. They have to take control straight away. Once you're detained you have no control.

Side effects

On the whole I've been pretty lucky with medication. It's been pretty good. I have had a rather large weight gain, but certainly my mood swings have mostly stabilised. I'm on a mood stabiliser, an antidepressant, a major tranquiliser . . . and I take anti-psychotics too . . . because I go psychotic sometimes. I often think someone is talking to me and for a long time I used to stand in the shopping centre and give people coloured stones and tell them that they would keep them safe. And you know, people would come up and take them! I would give them to my doctor too. It was considered a *nice* thing to do, but also insane! I haven't done anything like that for a long time.

Besides the weight gain, how did you find the side effects of the drugs?

Well when you first take the drugs you can look like a bit of a zombie and sleep a lot. Your eyes are glazed and starey. Once you get used to them it passes, but initially it can take a while.

I thought the positive effects outweighed the side effects until I got liver disease this year. The drugs are now irreversibly rotting my liver. The only option would be a liver transplant. I went yellow when it was really bad and I have a lot of pain in my gut. I spent ten days in hospital just recently because it was so inflamed. I can't have dairy products any more. I am very tired and I want to sleep a lot.

How do you feel about having such severe side effects?

It doesn't make me angry, but it certainly frustrates me. You have a mental illness, you take these drugs because they say that they are good for you and that they'll make you better. They may make the mental illness better, but they give you serious complications.

265

How have psychiatrists responded to these side effects?

They say that they knew that there was a remote chance that the drugs could rot my liver and unfortunately I was one of the unlucky ones. We're trying to lessen the dosages and see how I go.

I also notice that I am dry retching when I take my meds now, because I take a lot of other drugs as well . . . sometimes I just vomit them straight back up . . . I think psychologically I am saying to myself, 'I don't want to take these any more.' I'm going to have to find a way around it.

What are all the other drugs for?

I have Parkinson's Disease. It's settled in my legs and I've probably ignored it until this year. But I'm working at it now and that gives me a chance at a much better quality of life.

How long have you had Parkinson's?

Six years. I didn't really think that life was worth living after that one came down! But I got over it.

How did you get over it?

I don't know. It's just the way I am, I guess. I thought, 'Stuff it!' I also found out there was a guy high up in the mental-health field who has had Parkinson's for quite a while . . . he's got the shakes and everything. I thought, 'Well he's out there working and doing everything I want to do, so I am going to do the same.' So I did. I went to work.

A voice

I do contract work, giving talks to groups on depression. The fact that people took an interest in me as a good educator has been very valuable.

What has it given you?

Self-esteem. It taught me that I *did* have a voice and that I could use it . . . eventually . . . it didn't come straight away. Now I *can* use my voice to change things.

What does 'having a voice' mean for you?

It means that I'm no longer inhuman. It means I am no longer a 'non-person'. It means that I *do* count. It's also made me realise that people do respect me. It's given me a sense that I'm contributing. But it hasn't given me a reason to live on a permanent basis . . . though it does some of the time.

How did your work with them come about?

For some reason my key worker invited me to give a talk. They wanted some mental health consumers to talk about their experiences to service providers, health professionals and interested community workers. 'Okay, I'll do this,' I thought.

For years I had been terrified to even mention that I lived with mental illness, let alone had a husband who died from HIV/AIDS. There was such a stigma associated with both . . . I told them about my life since I was seventeen. My voice was shaking. I couldn't hold the paper. I told them how I'd become depressed and how that had developed into bipolar disorder. I told them about having two children who had died and then watching my husband die. And I had them crying. That deeply distressed me at the time, but that was a beginning of realising that I no longer had to be ashamed.

What was distressing about the fact that people cried?

I felt as though I'd given pain to others. I felt that you shouldn't give a talk that gives pain, you should give a talk that inspires people. I've since learnt that if people do cry, it's not necessarily bad pain – it's *good* pain. I've just recently started accepting that.

How do you see that 'good pain'?

It makes service providers think how they might change the way they talk to and treat people like me who are living with trauma and mental illness. It makes them think that they have to change the way they think and the words they speak.

Next week I am giving a talk to people who are doing a two-year counselling course. I'll probably tell them a few things about my life, to give them an idea of depression. I'll go through some statistics: that two out of five people will suffer from depression at some stage in their life, that by the year 2020 it will be the second highest disease affecting people in the world. Then I'll give them a snapshot of different approaches to depression that they can tap into: medication, cognitive therapy, ECT, there's so many now . . . I'll talk about the warning signs to look for in a one-on-one situation . . . to see if there is any suicidal ideation present for instance. I'll mention body movements like fidgeting and lack of eye contact. I'll talk about key words that depressed people might drop into a conversation in the hope that they will be picked up, and the fact that if you miss them that person might well go out and kill themselves.

Are these things which you exhibit when you are deeply depressed?

Well . . . I have a tendency to come over much stronger than I actually am, which can be a bit of a problem. People don't understand that I'm really suffering. I don't think I ever really gave any warning signs although I think my psychiatrist would pick up on things because he knows me really well.

For example?

I might just use a throw-away line like, 'I'm worthless'.

And then he might go through all the things I do. I might also avoid answering his questions. He might ask, 'How do you feel about suicide today?' and I'll go on to another subject. Then he will always bring me back.

You quoted some statistics to illustrate the high incidence of depression in society. How do you account for these?

Lifestyle for one. Families need two incomes. Life has changed dramatically and things are pretty stressful now. There's no relaxation any more. You don't see people just playing in the park.

I also think the media has a big impact. There's no point watching the news any more, because it really just stresses you out. I think it's a good idea to just forget about a lot of that stuff because you really can't do anything about it.

I also think a lot of people aren't like me when it comes to depression. They may be suicidal or depressed over smaller things, like 'My boyfriend broke up with me'. I think kids aren't educated well these days. They teach kids about sex but not how to cope with stressful situations, even *minor* stressful situations. I think people can be educated to know what stress is and the fact that it can come in many different forms. There's stress for a kid who misses the bus! Stress if you lose your job. I don't think they teach an awareness of the fact that stress is a part of life and life can't always be rosy. This would help enormously with regard to the high incidence of depression.

Of course at the moment the Welfare to Work[18] trouble is also going on. The government is going to take people

---

18 Welfare to Work is a $3.6 billion Federal Government initiative designed to move people off welfare and into work.

off the disability pension and make them go to work. This is going to devastate that population. There are an enormous number of people with mental illness who are simply not going to manage and I can see the suicide rate just going way up. At the moment about fifteen to twenty per cent of people with depression commit suicide. That's pretty high as it is.

Are you saying that there is no understanding of what it is like to live with depression?

None at all.

No reason

At present my life is relatively settled. I'm more at peace with myself than I've been in a long time. There's not so much turmoil. I'm still thinking constantly of death, but it's a little less, so perhaps I'm making progress with that. I'm always going to have battles but I hope that from now on they'll be more at the back of my mind than the front. Currently they're at the back.

What do you feel took you from almost killing yourself eighteen months ago to where you are now?

Good question. There wasn't really any startling revelation. I had some tests after I started having epileptic fits and I found out that I had probably sustained brain damage from the last suicide attempt. I had some more tests a bit later and there was also some brain damage that might be from Parkinson's. I thought, 'If I continue to attempt suicide, without actually achieving it, I will end up as a vegetable.' The thought of lying in a bed, unable to move my body but still conscious of everything going on, was a worry. I had also been unable to remember most of my hospitalisation and it worried me that I might have said things that under normal circumstances I wouldn't say. I think I made a conscious choice at that time that if I did it again, I would really have to get it right.

But there are other things as well. My contract work is very important. I also had a holiday in Queensland. It was cool. I relaxed. I did some fun things. All the stress got pushed away. It was lovely. I didn't realise how stressed I really was. It was my first holiday since my husband died, and I actually enjoyed it, which amazed me. There were moments when I thought it would be nice to have him there and hold his hand, but they were only moments. I also saw my daughter while I was away and it's had a big impact on my life that she's talking to me now ... like we used to be. I talked with her about everything and I saw my wonderful grandchildren.

... but I will always grieve for my children and my husband. I still struggle with the concept that it would be better for me to be with them than be here. I struggle every day of my life to think of something that will keep me here.

Do you feel there might be some reason as to why you *are* still here?

I suppose the people who saved me saw some reason as to why I should still be here. I think that life is just luck of the draw.

Do you have any sense of what the future might hold?

No. I don't have any sense of future. I haven't for a long time ... it got lost somewhere in the nine years my husband had HIV. I began to live day to day because that was all I could do. Each day was just so dramatic that I learnt not to project my thoughts into another day simply because I could not entertain the notion that it might be just as bad as the last. I quite simply *did not do it*. Even now I don't do it. If I get up in the morning, cool! Then I go and do what's in my diary. I even go to uni and study Behavioural Science and I still can't get any sense of future.

For what reason are you studying then?

No reason. I do it because I got high enough marks to do it.

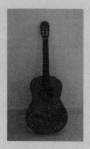

Meg

Meg is 27 years old. *'This is a photo of my guitar. Music has been very important to me for a long time. It has allowed me to disappear out of my anxious little world for a while and go somewhere else. It has been a stable thing in my life that is always there for me to come back to. Writing music is a way for me to express the things that other people don't necessarily understand.'*

On edge

I've always been quite an anxious person. Anxiety has flowed throughout my life in waves.

But it makes a lot of sense to me now why I have gone through life on edge. That's how I'd learnt to be. That's how I survived and that was all I knew.

My dad was a pretty heavy drinker. When he drank he was quite aggressive and if he wasn't drinking his nerves were really on edge. There were lots of arguments, lots of aggression and a lot of times that I felt completely out of control. I was always checking my environment, always waiting for things to go down and always preparing myself for the worst. It was like walking on eggshells the whole time. I was also very quiet and shy at school. I remember teachers saying, 'She's got a lot there, but her self-confidence is so low.' I learnt very quickly that my role was to stand back, be quiet and keep the peace.

There was nothing I could do to stop it all from happening.

Did you feel you should be able to do something?

Yeah I did. From the time I was very little I felt

responsible for looking after everyone and making sure they were all okay. I was the one who begged my parents to stop fighting. I was the one who consoled my younger siblings. Afterwards, I consoled my mother when she was crying in her room and then I sat on the back step with Dad who was drunk. I thought it would all fall apart without me.

I grew up in the country and it took me a long time before I could *leave* my home situation and move to the city, because in a way, it felt like I was leaving them for dead. I remember returning home one weekend, and realising what a truly awful environment it was to live in every day. I asked my mother, 'How can you live like this?'

Right through my time at uni I still hadn't identified the anxiety. I was going through thinking, 'There's something wrong with me. There's something weak about me. I'm not as strong as other people. I can't cope.'

I'd also been through *many* jobs. I always tried to put myself into management roles because I felt that then everyone would see that I *could* cope and *was* a successful person. I loved the first week of these jobs, because I didn't have to know anything. But after that there were always a million things running through my head. And then inevitably there was an expiry date on them: anywhere from three to seven months. By then I was completely burnt out and hated everyone and everything. Then I made an excuse, left and told a lie to another employer to get another job.

What sorts of excuses did you make?

Anything I could think of. 'I'd like to work more with people.' 'I'd like to work in a more personalised environment.' 'I'm also studying so I need less hours.' At one stage I had a very full-on job. I was shaking and could no longer talk to people, and so my solution was to go to a job in a very small store with very few customers. But I went just about crazy with boredom. Regardless of what I did, I still had this problem.

This problem
What was 'this problem'?

Generalised anxiety disorder. With the label it's given people think you're just a bit het up . . . a little bit anxious sometimes. But it's not like that at all. You have adrenalin pumping through your body 24 hours a day. There's very little respite from it. It affects your sleep. You shake. Your heart races. Your chest tightens. You can't breathe. It takes an incredible amount of energy *all* the time. In the mornings I woke up shaking – I called it 'shaking on the inside'. My entire body felt like it was crawling. I would think, 'Oh my god, I've got this awful feeling and I've got to go to work and talk to people! I'm not going to cope with the day!'

I got to a point at work that I couldn't even hold a pen. I couldn't disguise the fact that I was shaking uncontrollably. I was afraid people would think I was a drug addict or a psycho.

I also had panic attacks. I'd had them a few times at work and that was very embarrassing.

How long had you been having panic attacks?

. . . if I backtrack a little bit . . . during my year twelve exams I was under a fair amount of stress. I remember one day in particular was quite hot and I got this really strange feeling. It was like dissociation: I was there but I was not there. And then all of a sudden I just went bang. I lost consciousness and I had a seizure on the floor. I was taken to hospital and had lots of tests but the specialist eventually told me that the only thing he could put it down to was stress: 'You are incredibly stressed and your body has shut down.' I was put on an epilepsy drug for a year to stabilise things but I've never had a seizure since.

However, the feeling of going into a seizure is very similar to the start of both a really bad migraine and a panic attack. I'd had really bad migraines before, so I became very fearful of that particular feeling happening again. When I started having panic attacks, I'd go, 'Oh my god, I'm going to have another seizure!' I was forever waiting to have seizures. I don't think the panic attacks started because of the seizure but for a long time I associated the two.

Could you describe what happens during a panic attack?

First of all I might become really sensitive to the light. I might walk in somewhere or be standing somewhere and all of a sudden there's too much light. Fluoro lighting will do it for me. Large shopping centres where I'm amongst heaps of people will do it for me. Everything happens all at once and it starts to seem really over-whelming. Lights, space, people, noise. Then I'll think that I *have* to get out because there is so much horrible energy. I want to vomit or run or cry. Then you get the feeling that you are detached from your body. You're there, but you're not really there. Things aren't real. You're in space. There's space around you. You're out of your body. You're in another dimension or something. It's a funny feeling that's really hard to describe. It's a feeling of dissociation or detachment. Then I'll start to panic. My heart will start to race. I'll sweat. Shake. Start to hyperventilate. I'll feel like I'm going to pass out. I'll want to get down on the floor because then I can't fall anywhere and I won't feel quite so tall and big in the space. I won't necessarily think I'm going to die, but I'll certainly feel like everything is wrong and out of control. Often I'll burst into tears until it subsides.

I did learn ways of going through it that were a bit more socially acceptable than throwing myself down on the floor and crying. I might sit on a bench or go into a corner. In one of my jobs there was a hold room and I'd go in there. I'd just disappear. I'd think, 'I've got to hide and I've got to survive.' However, when it's a bad attack, there's nothing that you can do to hide it. It can feel quite humiliating.

Panic attacks usually come randomly when I'm a bit wound up. They're not associated with any specific fears. They're generally like a big explosion in the middle of all the anxiety. But I also remember times when I thought I wasn't wound up but I still panicked. I remember one day going to the lay-by department up the top of Myer. As I was walking up to the counter I got that awful detached feeling and I thought, 'Oh my god! I'm going to pass out! This is the last chance I have to tell someone that this is really serious!'

Was it your hope that someone would look after you if something did happen?

Yeah . . . It was really bizarre. I'd have these episodes when I'd think, 'I have to tell that person over there that this is about to happen to me.' And so I told the lady at the desk and she said, 'Just sit down over there.' So I sat down. Eventually I got up and got in the lift to go back down, and there was a family in there, and I thought, 'I have to tell them. I have to tell them that I'm about to fall over.' Eventually I got to the food court, sat down and drank some water and that helped. So I thought I must have been dehydrated . . . but of course I wasn't dehydrated. It was a panic attack. It wasn't the water that was helping me; it was simply sitting down and letting things settle. But I never thought, 'Oh this is just a panic attack!' Each time I thought it was potentially fatal.

Did you come to fear those attacks?

Yeah, I did. But I had two things going on at once. I had the fear of them because it is such an awful feeling. But sometimes I got to a point in my job where I'd feel so awful with the anxiety, that I *wanted* people around me to see how awful it was. I *wanted* to completely lose the plot.

This level of anxiety continued on and on until I had a few days off work. Then I relaxed and let go for a little while ... but it never lasted. The anxiety affected every opportunity that came up, it affected my relationships and it took a lot of my energy.

How did it affect your relationships?

It's interesting, because I recently spoke with my ex-partner who I'd been with for many years. I've done a lot of reflection on the role my anxiety played in sabotaging our relationship and I think it did more than I realised at the time. He didn't understand what was happening and nor did I. It was always put down to other things.

Like what?

He'd say, 'Oh you never want to do anything. You never want to mix with my friends. You're not adventurous.' They *were* things I wanted to be and do, but I felt I couldn't do them at the time and I didn't know why. In the end we just drew the conclusion that we were different.

So he didn't know you were anxious?

Not really. He knew I was nervy but neither of us knew that it was anxiety until we split and I worked out what was going on. Even then I don't think he fully understood what it was.

At the moment I feel incredibly angry because I realise how much the anxiety *did* influence things and I'm not able to go back and change that with him. He's moved on with someone else and I feel I've lost the opportunity to form a lifelong partnership.

How would you change it if you *could* go back?

I think I would be more willing to get out there and do different things: mix with different people and not be scared of being in a group. But I also wouldn't be so defensive. I made the assumption that I was a person who hated everything but it was completely the opposite. I wanted all those things for myself and I wanted to live a really full life but the anxiety and fear always held me back. Anxiety can play such a huge role in your life because you can't be how you would like to be.

What would enable you to do those things now?

Understanding what's anxiety and what's not. I would ask myself questions: 'Is this my anxiety talking or is this genuinely how I feel?' I couldn't distinguish between those two for a long time.

How *do* you distinguish?

I think you know in your gut. I think you know when you really want to do something but your anxiety is standing in the way; you know that you would feel regret if you didn't go ahead and do it.

Journal

When I was going through hard patches I wrote in my journal. My journal was somewhere to scream out all my feelings, to open up and write down whatever was in my head. Sometimes I wrote about what had happened, but other times it was feelings: anger, frustration. If I was really depressed I wrote words that didn't necessarily make sense. Sometimes it was just a scribble.

My journal had a different role to my music. It was a way of putting things in context; of getting things out of me so that I could look at them again. I now look at a lot of things I wrote and ask myself, 'My god, what was going on there?' I can see the patterns and the way I thought about things. I realise that although those feelings seemed very real to me at the time, I was actually a bit warped in my thinking.

Throughout my journals there are pages and pages of devising ways to run away: 'Today I'm going to put my notice in at work and then I'm taking a month off. I'm so tired and I've just had it. Once I set a date I won't feel so trapped. There'll be an end to this retail misery.' I'd have a grand plan and something to look forward to and then I'd feel a tiny bit of relief. Eventually I realised that those plans didn't really work.

The other day I read something I had written: 'I feel like I am living in this parallel universe to the rest of the world.' I got to the point where I felt completely detached and there was no way out of it.

Planting a seed

Understanding what was happening was very important and in the end it was the thing that relaxed me most.

I *knew* that past issues were affecting me but I didn't understand why the anxiety got as bad as it did. I went to counsellors and talked about some of the issues . . .

There was a counsellor I saw at uni and I explained everything to her. She didn't give me a really clear explanation but she did say something that was really important to me. She went right back to when I was little and said, 'You're suffering a lot of anxiety. Let's talk about where you've come from and what's happened in your life.'

She asked me about my mum. She asked me about my siblings. Then she asked me about my dad. I couldn't think of any words. She asked me again and then I launched into, 'Well he *drank* . . .' She asked me what *I* had done during all of this. And I told her. She leant right in, looked at me and said, 'So you were looking after everyone . . . but who was looking after you?' I just . . . burst into tears . . . She said that the anxiety I was feeling was about not feeling safe and never knowing what's coming up next. She told me that from an early age I'd learnt to live like that.

There was probably nothing there that I could have worked with, but it planted a seed. She pulled it all together for me. I went away and felt really angry, really sad, really resentful. It gave me something to think about.

But I continued on my search of, 'What do I do about this?'

I went to various GPs and asked, 'What's wrong with me?' I told them I was shaking and unable to cope. I wasn't able to describe it as well as I do now. There were times I walked in with my own conclusions: 'I'm taking the pill and my hormones are all over the place.' Naturally enough they suggested I try a different one. I really had no idea. But generally when women can't cope people *do* think it's the time of the month.

I went to one GP and told her, 'I'm incredibly anxious. I can't function. I can't work,' and she told me I was clinically depressed and needed antidepressants. Of *course* I was crying and depressed by the time I got in there, I'd had enough! She flipped it around the wrong way.

Did you take the antidepressants?

Not for very long. I stopped once I'd taken them long enough to experience the side effects. I felt that she was treating me for the wrong thing. The only thing the antidepressants did was to speed me up even more. My shaking and anxiety just took off. I remember going into a pharmacy and putting my hands out to show how much I was shaking. The pharmacist asked what I was taking, and she said, 'No! You need to cut the dose in half and go back to your doctor.' But rather than going back, I lost trust. I knew these people weren't listening to me and I knew I couldn't go back to them. I felt it had been my last hope and I completely lost faith.

Music

. . . and then one weekend . . . after I'd had a huge fight with some of my friends . . . I honestly felt like I didn't want to be here any more. I rang my mum and said, 'I don't want to go on with this any more.' I'd never said that before. I didn't have a plan to end my life but I felt that nobody understood and there was no light at the end of the tunnel. It was absolute despair. That weekend I picked up my guitar and wrote a song about being alone. I still connect with that song now. I still play it and can feel that same feeling . . . it's a really intense loneliness. It's not just, 'I'm bored and I'm lonely'. It's a feeling of complete detachment from everyone else. It's absolute loneliness.

Music is something I've always been passionate about. It's a means of expressing things in a way that makes sense to *me*. If I can get a lyric and refine it to the point that it captures the meaning of how I feel then it reflects the meaning back to me and helps me to understand myself.

Even as a child I'd go into my room and get out my

tape recorder. No matter what was going on I sat there and sang or played into it . . . lots of embarrassing songs! I was lucky that even when nothing was working in my life, I still had something I could turn to. It's always been a resource for me.

Creativity is almost the complete opposite of anxiety. Anxiety is about having lots and lots of things running around in your brain and experiencing an associated adrenalin rush. Anxiety tends to remove you from who you are and creativity is really the *essence* of who you are. When you can tap into creativity in some way, like I can with music, it keeps you connected with yourself. It's like a little channel that connects me straight to my centre. It's a place in my gut that holds the essence of who I am. I sort of light up.

Normalisation

I went to another doctor. And this time I was *so* lucky, because she said, 'You have anxiety. You have generalised anxiety disorder with panic attacks. This is *normal*. This is a *really* normal disorder. And given what you have told me about some of the things that have been happening in your life, it's no wonder!' She drew a little chart that illustrated the biological, the social and the environmental factors that influence anxiety.

How did her normalisation of it help you?

When you don't know what you have, you don't know where to go with it. When the doctor told me it had a name and was treatable, I felt I had a way to move forward. I felt relief. I felt someone had listened to me. That was really important.

What was important about someone listening to you?

I'd always felt like I was a fraud: 'This isn't really

happening. I'm just making it up. I'm a hypochondriac.'
If I did mention my anxiety to people they said, 'Oh
everyone gets a bit stressed.' They invalidated and dismissed
me. To see someone who told me my condition made
sense and that there were other people who suffered from
it too, put everything into context. It gave me hope. I no
longer felt so alone.

There are lots of people who hear you but they
don't really *listen*. They don't listen to the intensity of
what you're saying. They don't *know* it like you know
it. They don't feel any true empathy. People are just
polite and then it doesn't go any further. I think it's only
fellow anxiety sufferers who have been able to really
listen and feel the depths with me. You *need* that depth.
You need that spark to happen with someone else.

Anyway, that doctor booked me in for some sessions
with a psychologist who practised Cognitive Behavioural
Therapy. I went along to that, but I didn't really find
it all that helpful only because I don't think she was
actually doing CBT very well. There was no structure
and a lot of it was around breathing through panic
attacks . . . getting the oxygen/carbon-dioxide exchange
right. She was also trying to get me to set goals. She
was trying to get me to stay in my job. I suppose she
didn't want me to fall in a hole, but in reality I just *wanted*
to start again.

Around the same time however, I met someone
who had suffered with panic attacks and anxiety for
many years. He became a good friend and I owe him
a lot. I hadn't met anyone else who said, 'Hey I've been
through this and it's awful.' He was excellent because
he gave me a lot of advice about what to do when it
started to happen. And sometimes he actually put his
foot down with me and said, 'Do you want to stay here

or do you want to change? You're making a choice every single day about what's happening here.' He put the responsibility back on me while at the same time supporting me. He also listened to a lot of my garbage, 'Woe is me! I've cried all day!' But eventually he would say, 'I'm sick of hearing this. You do some things for yourself and stop just talking about it.' Although it still took me a while to catch on, he did plant a few seeds. He also gave me a lot of self-help books that were positive, motivational and helped me to recognise and *value* myself.

There was a really good book by Claire Weekes called *Self Help For Your Nerves*. It was about the actual anxiety and it gave techniques to let the panic flow past.

There was also a book called *Personal Mastery* by Julie T. Way. She does rebirthing and all that stuff. She talks a lot about the self and self-esteem.

I also read Fiona Harrold's *Be Your Own Life Coach*. It was about setting goals and believing that you can do things. It was also about changing your perspective and using things in your life positively. There was a chapter about being whoever you want to be. It wasn't about putting on a mask, it was about using your power to go out and get what you want. As someone with anxiety I was always thinking, 'What does that person think of me? They're looking at me. I'm a fraud. They're going to find out what I'm really about. Everyone's going to know and the show is going to be over.' I didn't take up opportunities because I thought I wasn't good enough and people would see through me. I thought I was all these ugly things underneath. She was saying that I wasn't a fraud and that people don't actually know as much as I think they know. She was giving me permission to believe in myself and be authentic. I thought, 'I can get away with a lot more than I ever let myself get away with. I don't have to be so hard on myself.'

I went along and picked out ideas from these books that worked for me and started to build up a bit of a toolbox. I started to look at how I was thinking, where that thinking was coming from but also how I was creating a lot if it myself.

What did you notice about the ways in which you had been thinking?

I was taking people's comments to heart.

Could you give an example?

'You're too sensitive.' That's something that people have *always* said to me. 'Oh, you're *so* sensitive!' In the past I would have seen it as a deficit. When someone says I'm sensitive now, I see it as a positive thing rather than as an attack. I accept that this is the sort of person I am. I say, 'Yes I *am* sensitive, and that's what makes me good at the things I'm good at.' There *are* instances when you have to be tougher, but it can also be a good thing to be sensitive.

This beautiful thing

It was only in my last job (*again* a management position) that I recognised that as well as everything else, I needed to give myself some time. I'd pushed and pushed myself and I needed time to reflect how I was coping with all of it. I approached the area manager and said I wanted to drop my position because I wasn't well enough. I didn't give excuses. I actually said that I was struggling in myself and needed to invest the time to get myself well. It was the first time I *hadn't* said, 'I can't do it because I'm incompetent and useless, so I'd better go.' It was the first time I'd been able to separate those two things.

While I was still at that last job I got in touch with an organisation that helps people with anxiety and asked if I could volunteer and they just happened to have a job available. It was a complete coincidence! By that stage I'd begun the recovery process. I knew what worked and what didn't and these were the strategies that were taught by the organisation. It reinforced the things I'd learnt about my own anxiety.

Was a pre-requisite for the job the fact that you had suffered from anxiety and panic attacks?

Yeah it was. I thought, 'My god, I can *use* this somewhere and I can help other people!' But although I'm now helping people as I did when I was young, I no longer lose my sense of self. Over time I have learnt that I can't afford to help people in the way I did in the past. If I do, I will eventually become emotionally bankrupt because there's nothing coming back in. I've learnt that I can continue to give and to help, but I need to do it on my own terms. I've learnt how to define my boundaries a little bit more.

How do you express those boundaries?

I definitely say 'no' more! But it's a process. I still come across situations where I give and give and give and I won't be aware of what's happening until it starts to take a toll on me. But that awareness *does* eventually come and the next time it happens I'm ready for it and I can say, 'I'm not doing that again. I'm not a bottomless pit.' I'm able to identify what is my responsibility and what isn't.

Could you describe your work a little more?

We do a lot of telephone support and we come into contact with a lot of people. To start off it was quite emotional because I got to experience the connection that people feel: 'Really? This is what's wrong with me?

And there are other people who have it? I'm not on my own? I'm not an alien?'

Because I've suffered from anxiety and panic attacks I can really connect with people. I feel so much empathy. I can *give so much* to other people. If anxiety hadn't been part of my life, this beautiful thing, this connection with people, wouldn't be in it! I wouldn't have this sense of achievement either. It's the sort of work I could go on doing forever and feel really fulfilled by.

Now I look on anxiety as a *blessing*! My work brings together all the things that happened in my life and makes sense of them. I've turned something that was *so* negative into something that's *such* a positive thing. And I've done it for myself. It's not like getting a brand new car and feeling good. It's a really *deep* thing.

Are you saying that you now see suffering as an opportunity to grow?

Oh yeah! I think without suffering you'd find it difficult to grow. It's difficult to grow if there's no reason to grow. If you stay in your safety zone you're never pushed to broaden your boundaries. Suffering is a horrible thing at the time but I think the pay-off for that is that you live a much fuller life. And a deeper life. And you can connect with other people better. There are many positive things that come out of suffering.

Looking back I also realise that you've got to trust people who have been through suffering when they say that things *will* get better and that it will all be worth it in the end. That's something that is really hard to do when you're in the middle of it all.

Do you still suffer with anxiety and panic attacks?

A lot of people ask, 'Have you recovered then?' I always say that it depends on what recovery means to you. I feel I *am* recovered, not because it never happens to me any more, but because I have a different perspective. It doesn't affect me like it used to. I can understand and intervene in the cycle of anxiety when it happens.

I now think of things in terms of strategies. I'm able to break things down into bite-size pieces so that they're really not such a big deal. Instead of feeling overwhelmed, I *manage* what's going on. 'Okay, so this is happening. So what can I do about it? Okay these are the things I can do and these are the things I can't do.'

For example, a little while ago I'd been sleeping badly because there were a lot of stressful things going on. I woke up one morning and I was sitting at the table eating breakfast. I was trying to pick up my cup of tea and I was shaking. In the past I would have gone, 'I can't cope. Look at me. This is awful!' But I sat there and said to my housemate, 'Oh I've got the shakes. Look at my hand. But that's okay because there have been a lot of stressful things in my life lately. It's no wonder because I'm pretty tired.' I normalised it and put it into a context. I didn't give it power and it didn't take over. I didn't catastrophise. Instead of running from it and avoiding it, I looked it in the eye.

I've come a long way and I am actually a strong person.

Trevor

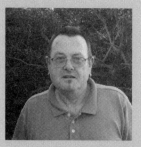

Trevor is 57 years old. He was born in England and moved to Australia in 1972. He describes himself as a mental health consumer, systems advocate, community and mental health consumer representative, health activist, experiential educator and peer support promoter. *'My birthday is on the 10th October and that is World Mental Health day. I think I must have been destined to take the path that I have! . . . that's just a joke!'*

My mental health journey commenced in England in 1964 when I was sixteen. A young lady broke up with me and I was absolutely devastated. I took a massive dose of aspirin to kill myself. I suppose it was the standard knee-jerk reaction that some young men have.

You didn't feel you had any other way of coping with the situation?

No. No way to cope with it. I probably took about 100 aspirin . . . I was found by a friend wandering in the vicinity of my house. I was in a very confused state and he took me home. My mum realised what I had done and she called an ambulance. They took me off to hospital, I had my stomach pumped . . . and I lived to tell the story. I did see a psychiatrist once at the hospital, but he was absolutely useless. The only thing he asked me was what I wanted to do when I left school. I told him that I wanted to join the merchant navy so that I could leave home. And he said, 'Well that's a good idea.' And so I did.

But it actually wasn't a good idea, because I had a death wish. At night I'd get drunk, and I'd want to jump over the side of the ship.

Was that death wish an ongoing consequence of the relationship ending?

On reflection it was a lot deeper than that. As a single young man I always sought a permanent relationship. I was never one for one-night stands.

I was in the merchant navy for about three years. And then when I was nineteen, while I was still in the merchant navy, I had a serious car accident that nearly killed me. The car accident really brought me back down to earth with a big thump. It gave me a big shock. It changed my attitude.

Did that shock bring a new appreciation of life?

I don't know that I have *ever* appreciated life! I just realised that the merchant navy wasn't good for me, because I didn't have a lot of self-discipline and the booze was too easy to come by. And in any case I was advised not to go back to sea because the car accident had left me with a hole in my skull from a brain operation.

But while I was in the process of recovering from these injuries I met my wife and I began to settle down. I was nineteen and she was sixteen. In 1972, after two years of marriage, we came to Australia. The effects of the depression just seemed to disappear. The death wish went away. And everything was hunky-dory . . .

But when I was 47, things changed. I was once again plagued by suicidal ideation. I had constant thoughts of suicide.

They started out of the blue?

Yes . . . but on reflection, my wife and I realised that the change was actually seven years in the making.

I was working in the superannuation, investment and

life insurance industry which was very goal oriented. I was quite successful at it and won a trip to a sales conference in Rio de Janeiro. I really wanted to go there, because I'd been there in '66 when I was in the merchant navy and I wanted to see how much it had changed. I achieved that goal, but after I came back I was lost and couldn't get motivated again. I think that was the start of my downhill journey. Then my wife had her car stolen and that seemed to really upset me. I also remember driving along with her one day and having a feeling that we were going to go bankrupt. There was no particular reason for this, because business was really good.

After that, I started to get thoughts of suicide. I went to work for long hours but I wasn't doing any work. My job involved talking to people but I couldn't even pick up the phone. Then I went with my wife to my GP because I knew that I needed some professional help. But rather than admit that I was suicidal, I complained to the doctor about a pain under my ribs on the left-hand side. He diagnosed me as having stress and gave me a referral to a GP who specialised in counselling. Well I'm a *bloke*, and I didn't want to go to counselling. That referral sat on my desk for a further three months until things got worse and worse . . . eventually I knew that I had to bite the bullet and go and see this guy.

Could you describe this 'worse and worse'?

My work was building up and it was getting out of control. I couldn't answer the phone. I'd lost interest in life. I'd become 'nothing' inside. Void. I could still tell a joke. I could still appear happy on the outside, but the poor little bugger on the inside was very depressed. I'm still like that today, but I just don't have the suicidality.

You went to see the counsellor . . .

Yes. Stuff about my past came up . . .

My father died when I was four and I don't remember ever grieving. I do remember that my mother grieved twice a year because two of her husbands had died. My mother was a woman who displayed her emotions to the full and because I am a male, I didn't approve. When I was nine or ten, because I had no dad, I used to play truant from school and lead her a merry dance. She used to get really upset and hit me with a leather dog lead. Then she would break down in tears and say, 'It hurts me more than it hurts you.' That had such an impression on my life. I believe my mum did a good job of bringing me up on her own, but I felt unloved. I had a half-sister who lived with us. She was eight years older than me and she was the apple of my mother's eye. She was more intelligent than I was, she did better at school . . . and that totally pissed me off. When my mother died in 1992, even though I spent the last four days with her in hospital, I never shed a tear.

My wife came with me to one of the interviews with the counsellor and at one stage she started to cry because of the impact my suicidality was having on her. I must have indicated in some way that I didn't approve of her crying, because he pointed out that it was quite alright for her to cry. I remember telling the counsellor that I couldn't stand women crying and that if my wife cried I would simply walk out of the room . . . I must have been a real bugger to live with. That's when I realised that I'd always had this big hang-up about people crying and that I would always blame myself for any female that cried . . . I'm different now . . . my wife can cry away to her heart's content if she wants! But *I'm* still unable to cry. I can't cry.

The mental health service believes that depression is

a chemical imbalance in the brain and that it can be either endogenous (created by an internal cause) or exogenous (created by the environment). I think the endogenous bit is a lifetime of things locked away inside . . . all that baggage was locked away behind my steel shutters and had a lifelong effect on me.

In any case this counsellor gave me hypnotherapy twice and on the second occasion, because I'd built up some trust with him, I told him I was suicidal. He put me on an antidepressant that completely zonked me out and I had to stop working. As an antidepressant it didn't help me at all. This particular antidepressant is known among consumers as the 'suicide pill', because it actually exacerbates people's suicidality. And that's what it did to me. I felt even more suicidal. And as a result the GP eventually referred me to a psychiatrist. And that's when it started . . .

'It'?

My journey . . . my journey through the depressive illness.

The first psychiatrist I saw asked me to tell him about my life and the only thing I could relate to him was the fact that people in my family had died. I couldn't think of anything positive. In reality I lived in a very supportive environment with two beautiful adult children, but I could only relate the deaths in my family. That enabled him to very quickly assess that I had a major affective disorder. He was actually a bit weird though, because he didn't prescribe medication. It wasn't that he didn't believe in it, it was just that he wouldn't prescribe it. He'd send me to another psychiatrist for my medication. I called him my 'alternative psychiatrist'.

Why didn't he prescribe medication?

I've no idea. It was probably some personal point of

view. Perhaps the fact that he was what they call a 'family' psychiatrist (he worked with families) had something to do with it. In any case I was unable to have any sort of therapeutic relationship with him, because he wanted me to do things that I simply couldn't do. He'd say, 'Imagine that you are an ant in your chest.' And I'd say, 'I can't. This is *me* right now, sitting on your couch.' Then he'd say, 'Well if you're not going to comply with what I'm asking ...' I would tell him that it wasn't that I didn't want to comply but that I was unable to. I didn't have a vision like that.

I was seeing him every week, but I never wanted to go there. We'd always end up arguing and arguments only made the depression worse. I probably saw him for about six months ... in the end I told him that I wanted to find somebody else. He agreed with me completely. However, he strongly recommended that I participate in a group therapy weekend that he was running. There were seven of us. That was horrendous.

In what way?

We had to do role plays and games and I just didn't want to play. He had the whole group imagining that they were on a space ship in outer space. Everybody was jumping from cushion to cushion. It was good for making the group come together but I had great difficulty with my imagination at that time. I was robbed of my imagination and I just couldn't participate. I couldn't play. I'd sit in the corner and frown.

I wrote a poem about the people in the group, with a verse devoted to each. This is what I wrote about myself:

Trevor the Iceman he came on his own,
Because inside him there is no one home.

I signed it, 'Trevor – he who looks inside but has yet to see'.

What was the overall objective of the group?

Well the fact is that the other six, even the blokes, all ended up crying at some stage. They were obviously able to release something. Good luck to them, but I couldn't do that. I probably hadn't cried since I was sixteen. Anyway, that cost me $400 and on the pension, that's pretty hard.

This psychiatrist also recommended a change of medications. I was admitted to a public psychiatric ward for what they call a 'medication washout' – seven days with no medication – during which time they monitored me. I was really bloody depressed and suicidal and after two days on the ward a psychiatrist interviewed me and it was hate at first sight. This man thought he was God's gift to women. He thought he was Adonis! I'd only just started to grow my hair longer and had earrings put in my left ear, and he said to me, 'Men of your age do *not* have long hair and they certainly don't wear earrings.' I was also wearing a T-shirt that I'd been given by friends who had just returned from San Francisco. It read, 'ALCATRAZ PSYCH WARD OUTPATIENT'. I think that really fired him up. He felt that wearing such a T-shirt in the psychiatric ward was very poor custom. He certainly had no sense of humour.

Anyway, he decided in the ten-minute interview that I did not have depression, that I was not suicidal, and that instead I had a narcissistic personality disorder. He said I was to go home, stop taking the medication and contact my psychiatrist. He discharged me. I tried to hang myself two days later.

Back in '95, if there was a diagnosis of personality disorder, it was very convenient, because they could throw you out of hospital. They had no time for you because it wasn't considered a serious mental illness. Even now, there are still difficulties in getting assistance for people diagnosed with a personality disorder, but in those days they were just left to their own devices.

Six months after that, I became very angry about what had occurred because it could have cost me my life. I researched the diagnostic criteria for narcissistic personality disorder from the DSM IV[19] and there were nine of them. I could see that on that day I had displayed four of those criteria, but that psychiatrist had actually displayed *seven* of them!

I wrote a series of six poems about the incident and one of them I entitled *Dr So-and-so – god with a little 'g'.* This did me wonders!

> Dr So-and-so, the head honcho psych,
> Wanted to assess my personal strife . . .
> Empathy lacking, none did I see,
> The bastard sent me home for tea.
> There'll be no pills for you to take,
> If you suicide, that's your mistake.
> My hands are clean, says 'god' to me,
> I've had my training, don't you see . . .

I actually delivered those poems to his rooms in an envelope and apparently, I was told later, when he opened them he immediately phoned the mental health service to find out if I was dangerous! There was no threat in them whatsoever.

You mentioned that two days after the incident you tried to hang yourself.

---

19 Diagnostic and Statistical Manual of Mental Disorders.

Yes. I felt completely abandoned by the public health service that was meant to be there to assist me. Not only that, I was at home alone and I was drinking. I tried to phone Lifeline eighteen times and I was never connected. And then in desperation I tried to pull the plug. I had the stool and the rope up over the pergola, the rope around my neck . . .

Something stopped you?

I think perhaps it was self-preservation. The body doesn't want to die even if your head does.

When I realised what I was doing, I drove myself to the local hospital. I was really drunk. At that stage you couldn't get into the psych ward of the local hospital without first being admitted at the psychiatric hospital (it's changed now). The doctor in the emergency department said, 'I'll get you a cab down to the psychiatric hospital.' I told him that I didn't have the money for a cab and that I would drive myself. And so I did! I got there at two in the morning and thankfully I didn't hit anything on the way. I was assessed by about six different people. They breathalysed me, gave me breakfast and then breathalysed me again. Then they said I could be admitted to the local hospital and that I could drive myself back over there! And even more bizarre was the fact that I was put back in that ward under the same psychiatrist . . . the Adonis fellow . . . for a further eleven days.

On discharge from that ward, my wife and I were interviewed by him, to make sure I was happy to be going home, and as I was walked out of his office door he said to me, 'Aahhh . . . I knew you wouldn't commit suicide.'

I later learned that this psychiatrist was newly qualified. I think psychiatrists need to bear in mind, particularly when they are newly qualified, that they don't have a lot of experience with people and their behaviours.

It is also impossible to form any close relationships with psychiatrists in the public system because you don't see them often enough.

A couple of years later I was back in the same ward. I still suffered from depression and suicidal ideation. My wife and I had had some words of disagreement. I stormed out of the house and drove my car up to a hill with the intention of driving off. I sat up there for hours, contemplating killing myself, but I didn't. Eventually I drove myself to hospital and got admitted.

During my hospitalisation someone said to me that having a mental illness could be likened to a man who has had his third heart attack. After the first heart attack, friends and relatives rally around; there's lots and lots of support. Second heart attack comes along and family and *some* friends are still supportive. But after the third heart attack, the 'not again!' syndrome sets in and you'll have very few people supporting you apart from your immediate family. I thought that was a good analogy.

Had you continued to be depressed over those two years?

Yes. The whole time. And I was medicated the whole time. I was on various antidepressants. In the first four-and-a-half years I went through seven antidepressants. Some didn't work. Others might initially work but then the benefits would wear off, so that eventually I would only have side effects. I wrote a poem about the side effects of one particular drug, and I listed sleep disturbance, anxiety, dizziness, blurred vision, diarrhoea, dry mouth and confusion.

I continued to see a private psychiatrist once a month as a consumer of the local public mental health team. I was really fortunate, because when I was really unwell

I also had a key worker who visited me at home once a week. A couple of times when I was in dire straits, I did phone her and fortunately she had the time to visit. And that assisted me.

In what way?

When I'm in a crisis and if I'm suicidal I need to speak to somebody face to face. It's no good talking to them on the phone. It isn't effective. Face to face gives you some sort of instant relief. Sometimes if I was in crisis I found that even if I could just go and sit in the waiting room of the mental health services office, I received a degree of relief. I still needed to talk to someone . . . but it was a place of safety.

The fact of seeing a psychiatrist once a month, on its own, never gave you that sense of safety and contact?

No. It was the access to the key worker that was so important . . . and you would never get psychiatrists to visit you!

What was the key worker by profession?

Well I had a number of them over the years. They were part of a multi-disciplinary team. Initially they were mental health nurses, but you might also have a social worker, an occupational therapist or a psychologist.

Did the key workers give you therapy or simply manage crises?

Well I was very fortunate that one of my key workers was the team leader of the community mental health clinic and also a psychologist. I had a good therapeutic relationship with him, as well as a working relationship (when I put on my mental health consumer representative hat – we never confused the two). The therapy was a talking therapy, but don't ask me what it was. I was once given some information on Cognitive Behaviour Therapy and that stuff frightened the shit out of me. It seemed to highlight all the things that I already saw as being wrong with me: my character, my thoughts, my faulty thinking. The whole depression thing is wrapped up in self-hate and self-blame and so it left me feeling even more depressed; it made me despise myself even more. I explained this to the key worker . . . and perhaps in his own subtle way there was some CBT, but it wasn't rigid. The therapy was successful, though very lengthy, and I gradually built up skills and resilience to cope with my symptoms.

For instance?

For instance, when I was very depressed I would catastrophise dramatically and I would almost immediately start to think of suicide. This could happen over as small an event as my wife changing the tone of her voice. But I wish to point out that although to the outer world it may be seen as catastrophising, to the person who is suffering it *really* is drastic and dramatic. Talking with the psychologist I learnt to recognise the precursors and how to cope with them. Gradually I needed less and less contact and after four-and-a-half years I seemed to turn a corner. I realised that I was self-managing my illness and that I'd lost the compulsion to see a key worker, even on a monthly basis.

You mention that you had a working, as well as therapeutic, relationship with your key worker. How did you come to be a consumer representative?

The impetus came from that incident with that Adonis fellow and the fact that I was discharged with a well-and-truly incorrect diagnosis. That whole incident could have damaged me for life with regard to my feelings towards the mental health service or it could have cost me my life. I thought that nobody else should have to go through the same thing; I wanted to do something about it. I joined the newly formed local consumer advisory group and we still meet once a month. We advise the mental health service on consumer and carer issues. As a group we do systemic advocacy.

What do you mean by systemic advocacy?

Encouraging or advocating for the mental health service to change its system to suit consumers and carers. The first bit of systems advocacy that I was involved with was at a psychiatric clinic. The safety glass in the office was very consumer/user unfriendly. The office floor for the staff was higher than the waiting-room floor and the speaking slits in the glass were not in the right place for either side to talk with one another with a degree of comfort. The consumers had to either be three feet or seven feet tall to speak through the glass. I surveyed other consumers and they agreed with me. I advocated for the safety glass to be changed. That was the first thing. It wasn't life shattering, but it made it easier for people to use the service.

Did you feel that the fact that the staff floor was higher than the consumer floor, was an issue with regard to inequity?

Since the onset of my mental illness I have lost the pedestal effect of doctors and professors. Everyone who at one stage I would have thought of as 'better' than me, has come down to my level. I respect them for their specialisation, but I also expect respect from them for what I do. I am also an expert in my field.

That's a very big leap from the times you describe yourself as filled with self-hate and self-blame. How did that change come about?

I'm not sure exactly how that came about. I assume that my long-term representation on service provider committees helped me to relearn many of the life skills I lost through the severe clinical depression. I have talked with everyone from the professor of psychiatry at the major hospital, to the director of mental health services in the state, to politicians, to service providers in general . . .

And do you find that they indeed give you that respect?

Yes I do . . . perhaps some are only paying lip-service, but nobody's actually made it obvious without me letting them know that I don't approve.

How would you let someone know that you don't approve?

In 1997, I telephoned a senior project officer in the mental health unit in the Department of Human Services. I'd heard that he was having a meeting with a non-government organisation around supporting mental health consumers. I said to him, 'You need to have a consumer on that committee, because you can't go talking about supporting consumers without consumer representation.' He said to me, 'Trevor, we only have important people on that committee.' I replied that I considered myself to be *very* important. I still work with that guy and he doesn't have that attitude any more.

How did he respond at the time?

I think he was a bit dumbfounded! . . . and obviously for a while he was not my favourite service provider . . . but things have changed since '97. I'd like to think that there aren't too many people left who think like that. Within the local mental health service, consumer representation works very well because we've always had support from *the* senior person/people. Then along with the support from a hardcore group of key workers, it can all happen from the ground up.

Was consumer representation initiated by consumers?

No. The consumer movement within the regional mental health service was actually started by B . . . who was a psychiatrist. At the time he was the director and it was his idea to form a consumer advisory group. He encouraged some social workers to bring together a group of consumers.

What was he hoping to achieve?

To change the service through consumer and carer input, and I believe that works.

When I initially joined the regional advisory group in August 1996, it seemed that nobody (consumers, carers or service providers) knew what we were supposed to do. But by November we were asked to sit on our first committee, and I think we had six consumers . . . it was too many, but it was a good grounding. The director of the mental health service and all the other bigwigs were on this committee. Most consumers were reluctant to talk, but I soon got the hang of it . . . and these days there's no shutting me up! The two consumer advisory groups are a big part of my life now.

In these working committees they usually have an item that requires consumer/carer input, and I suppose that's their way of asking for our help. I am someone who has input anyway. If I see a way, for instance, of saving money, I will suggest it.

If you look at your work as a whole, what would you say is your fundamental aim?

To keep the consumer profile in front of the committees so that the mental health service can't forget we're there. When I first joined the regional advisory group I said to B . . ., 'What's the point of this consumer representation?' And he said to me, 'Trevor, it's to keep the bastards honest.' And I think that's probably it. We're there to promote our point of view and if things are wrong, advocate for change.

If it's to keep 'the bastards honest', how are the bastards dishonest?

That's just a phrase! . . . but in 1999, for instance, there was a complaint from a female consumer who had been in a lockup ward in the psychiatric hospital. They had no sanitary disposal unit. The poor woman had her period and had to leave the sanitary pad on the floor. That meant that staff had to come along and dispose of it. I can understand that happening in 1899, but not in 1999! They probably couldn't have had those bins with the chemicals in them, but what's wrong with a paper bag? This had been going on for decades. That practice was changed.

So basically it is about treating consumers like human beings.

Yes. Some mental health professionals don't treat consumers very well. They have an attitude problem that they need to change. And we need to help them do that. If I get a complaint about an individual worker, I will actually approach their team leader, but not in an accusing way. The way that I approach this kind of advocacy is that it's always the fault of the system. If you have a mental health nurse who has worked at a psychiatric hospital for the past 30 years, and has a bad attitude towards consumers, it actually isn't their fault. It's the fault of the system, and the fact that perhaps that person has missed out on training. 'The system' is a good scapegoat; that's worked brilliantly for the past nine years.

And do you personally believe that the system is always to blame?

Yes, of course the system is to blame, because even if that nurse hadn't been there for 30 years, if they have an attitude problem, well then they shouldn't have had the job in the first place! That's why I believe it's so important to have consumers on staff selection panels. I have been on some very senior staff selection panels, but it doesn't happen at the junior level. In my local area consumers are asked to provide a representative on staff selection panels for team leader and above. We've been doing that since 1998. I was on the staff selection panel for the current director for the state.

Do you have equal say?

Oh yes!

And what criteria do you use?

An awareness of consumers and carers; who they are and where they're coming from. A knowledge of recovery style services; not being reliant on clinical models alone. An understanding that in the recovery model people need to be treated holistically, not merely as a diagnosis.

What do you mean by holistically?

One of my major issues with the mental health service is that for two years, from '95 to '97, I advocated very strongly for my local community mental health team to talk with my wife about the likely progression of my depressive illness. I constantly met with a brick wall: 'We don't talk to families.' It is so important to involve every-body. It actually happens now. Even friends can be involved in discussions.

There is more to me than just depression. When I was seriously ill for four-and-a-half years they treated only the depression. Nothing else. There was no other generic health and lifestyle education and there was no peer or non-clinical support. I was reliant on the mental health service. After I turned the corner, I told the team leader, who was also my key worker, that I was quite critical of the treatment I had received. I believe that four-and-a-half years is too long. I wondered what they could have done to get me to where I was in a shorter space of time. I came up with the idea that they had only treated depression. They hadn't treated me holistically. They hadn't looked at my life as a whole.

You mentioned a recovery style and opposed it to the clinical model. Could you tell me a little more about this?

A recovery focus is one in which the consumer is encouraged to regain their life. It is something like the Lorig Chronic Disease Self-Management Education Model, which is a six-week generic health and life style education program. Kate Lorig is a nurse from Stanford University.

That model has been well-developed and well-recognised worldwide as an effective education program. I felt that it was applicable to mental health because in my experience mental illness had robbed me of all the skills that I had. I had become a non-person. I would read a sentence but I couldn't make sense of it. I could read things 90 times and yet it would not make any difference. I was fortunate that my wife was very supportive, but other single males with depression become unkempt, unclean and don't feed themselves. People need to relearn basic living skills.

How would you implement that?

It's already been done. Between 2002 and 2003 I had the idea of a Chronic Disease Self-Management Mental Health Project. It developed from my initial ideas of what was missing from my treatment. We actually got funding from the Department of Human Services to develop this over an eighteen-month period. We based it on the Lorig model. It is preferably delivered by peer educators.

We trialed it on consumers with a serious mental illness who either have a dual diagnosis of a physical illness or the chance of developing one. (Though actually everyone with a diagnosis of mental illness has a chance of developing a physical illness.) I was one of the co-educators. Consumers were recruited by key workers. It was run over a six-week period for two-and-a-half hours a week.

What issues did you address?

Exercise, healthy eating, relaxation, being aware of your illness (your precursors and stressors) and also how to talk with your treating team. Some professionals have forgotten that they have a duty of care to tell their patients about the pros and cons of taking medication for instance. It's teaching consumers to be assertive, to take the opportunity to ask questions and to know that anything that they might want to discuss is important. Consumers have a right to have a say and be listened to . . . it was a really great course. We were able to run two groups with a total of 36 consumers and our dropout rate was very low. Because it was the first time in the world that it had been trialed with mental health consumers, we had a clinician sitting in just in case anything went wrong. But nothing went wrong.

Was the group successful?

Absolutely. One of the very strong things about the model is that it uses action plans to start people doing things. We'd meet and people would say what their action plan for the next week was. Because of group dynamics people felt obliged to do what they said they were going to do. There was also encouragement and understanding of difficulties from within the group.

One woman who came to the group was very

depressed: shoulders down, head down. The first week she volunteered no information though participated if asked. Her action plan was to go to the library and borrow a book on wood burning art. The second week she was an entirely different person: erect, head up. She started to offer advice to other participants. Fourteen months later I went to interview her and her artwork was magnificent! She said she still uses her action plans on a daily basis in order to get something done.

This morning there was an article in the paper that stated that the mental health system in Australia is in a very poor state. Do you agree with this?

I believe that mental health professionals at the coalface are doing the best job they can do in a very under-resourced situation. It's *funding* that's the problem. When it comes down to individual service delivery, people do their best. The majority of mental health professionals don't go to work to *damage* people! They don't go to work and think, 'Well I might go and upset a consumer today!'

However, because of under-funding there is a deficiency of *community* mental health services. In my local clinic, although the services have increased since 1995 when I became a client/patient/consumer, the actual number of full-time employees has gone backwards. They actually have *fewer* staff to service a population that's probably three times greater than it was in 1995. You can be critical of the service because it can't provide the care that's required, but it isn't *their* fault.

In that same article it quotes an MP as saying, that if you have a family member with a mental illness, then there is nowhere to go.

Well, you have to know *where* to go.

Do you believe that people know where to go?

Generally not.

Where *should* people go?

As a consumer you can contact consumer groups. Carers can contact carer groups.

What if a consumer is in a crisis?

Well then you phone ACIS[20] . . . but you have to actually make out that you have a razor at your throat and you're just about to die . . . and then you'll get a service.

Are you saying that you have to act in a catastrophic way in order to get some care?

Yes. Yes. Yes.

One of the major problems I initially had in trying to get help was that I can be very rational. I have no emotions. I suppose the pain inside could be viewed as an emotion, but for me there was just an overwhelming depression and self-hate. And I present too well. It's difficult to get a service if you present really well because it doesn't seem as if you need help. And the fact is that you really don't *want* to present to someone that you're mentally unwell and you want to die!

So if you present well and say in a reasonably calm voice, 'I'm desperately unwell,' they don't listen to you?

That's right. I strongly believe that ACIS, being the crisis unit in SA, should actually tell consumers who are suicidal to phone Lifeline, because they'll get a bloody better service! Lifeline gives you counselling even if it's only over the phone. If you ring them and say that you're feeling suicidal, that's of great concern to them.

---

20 Assessment and Crisis Intervention Service (SA). In other states: Crisis Service in NSW, Crisis Assessment and Treatment Service (CAT) in Victoria and ACT, Mobile Intensive Support Team (MIT) in Queensland, Psychiatric Emergency Team (PET) in WA, On-Call Team in NT.

ACIS doesn't offer a crisis *counselling* service. It is a crisis mental health service *triage*. They assess the risk over the phone and manage the situation. It may depend on the individual, but it isn't in their mandate to talk to you. If you phone up and say you're suicidal (and this happens with *all* the crisis teams around Australia) they tend to give very glib remarks that sound uncaring: 'Why don't you make a cup of tea? Why don't you do the gardening? Why don't you go for a walk around the block?' How's that going to help you when you frickin' want to die? Obviously there are also some very good people on the end of the phone but there are also some very bad ones.

What does it do for a person in crisis when they're told to go and do the gardening?

Well this actually happened to me, and I said, 'I hate fucking gardening!' . . . and I hung up. It wasn't helpful! If I'm in a crisis and I'm feeling suicidal, I need to speak to someone face to face . . .

I think it's so important for professionals to *listen*. This is just as true of life as it is of psychiatry – *people need to learn to listen!* They would learn a lot more by just listening. Men are dreadfully bad at listening. They just tend to give solutions and that's not necessarily what people in crisis want. Whatever the consumer or patient says is *right* and the professional needs to be trained to pick up signs or certain words or whatever.

In my work as a consumer consultant in the psychiatric ward at the hospital, I believe my most important assets are that I have big ears for good listening, broad shoulders to carry a burden, and I am non-judgemental. I approach people as fellow human beings. That's what consumers want.

Early on you said that it's impossible to form a

close relationship with psychiatrists in the public system because you don't see them often enough.

You can't form a relationship with a psychiatric registrar who is only there for six months. The public mental health service is a *teaching* mental health service. It's the only way for psychiatric registrars or psychiatrists-in-training to learn their trade: how to diagnose and treat people. The public system, particularly the hospitals, couldn't exist without the registrars.

So if the mental health system is used as a teaching apparatus, are there any psychiatrists who actually stay for longer than six months?

Well obviously these registrars work under senior consultant psychiatrists who oversee what they do . . . and *they* stay longer than six months . . . and people are always entitled to a second opinion, though I don't think anyone realises that.

I believe that if you can't have a therapeutic relationship with a psychiatric registrar, you're beating your head against a brick wall. That's why I see a psychiatrist privately . . . but of course there is generally a co-payment. There are a few who bulk-bill, but they are few and far between and obviously they'd be overloaded.

How often do you see your private psychiatrist?

Monthly. I have a good therapeutic relationship with him, and he's been my psychiatrist since '96.

Do you feel that is the only option available for people who wish to see a psychiatrist regularly?

Yes it is.

Do people know that?

I don't think they do. The majority of consumers on the disability support pension wouldn't be able to find the extra money to see a private psychiatrist.

At the beginning of the interview you said that

you're not sure that you have ever appreciated life? Is that still true?

Although I function very well, I still have depression. It is controlled by medication, but I feel quite sure that if I had any sort of trauma in my life, it could re-emerge very rapidly.

I generally live day by day and I don't see a future for myself beyond today. I don't have any hopes or dreams.

... even though you're actively involved in the consumer mental health movement, and you seem quite passionate about your activities ... ?

... but I *expect* myself to do that. I just expect that I'm able to do that. I do what I do because it needs to be done.

I take one day at a time. In my previous life I had hopes and dreams and things like that ... but they seem to have vanished ... I couldn't say to you what I plan to do in two years' time. My life just happens.

Author's postscript

Shortly after I completed this interview, Trevor was diagnosed with bowel cancer. He passed away on 15 November 2006. His funeral was a very fitting celebration of his life. Trevor often said that cancer was somewhat similar to mental illness: its mere mention left people uneasy and unsure as to what to say.

In my interview, Trevor spoke a number of times of his inability to cry and also his discomfort when other people cried:

> ... *I'm* still unable to cry. I can't cry ... all that baggage was locked away behind my steel shutters and had a lifelong effect on me.

On 10 October 2006, approximately five weeks before his death, Trevor was announced as the winner of the 2006 Dr Margaret Tobin Award for Excellence in Mental Health in the category Consumer/Carer/Volunteer. This public acknowledgment of his achievements affected him deeply. He had previously sat on the panel for these awards and was well aware of the rigorous selection criteria involved.

I had a conversation with Trevor approximately two weeks before his death and the thing he most wished me to recount in this postscript was the fact that on receiving this award, he had cried.

Glenda

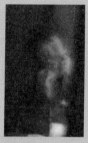

Glenda is 48 years old and has lived with spinal muscular atrophy from birth. She enjoys living on her own. Her garden is very old and she hopes one day to restore it to its original condition. She has three cats and calls them 'my kids'. She has always barracked for the underdog whether that be the St Kilda football team or an injured animal. Although she likes going out, she isn't able to do that as much as she used to. She has always enjoyed painting and drawing, but because of her increasingly limited strength, she now pursues her art through the use of digital camera and computer technology. *'This photo was spontaneous. It was as though I snuck up on myself. My eyes shine out even though they are vague and dim and the photo is blurred. I have always hated my skinniness and yet in this photo I feel my long thin fingers represent who I am with great beauty.'*

The first time I got depressed I was about fourteen. I lived in the country and I had been sent down to a crippled children's home in the city for three months of physiotherapy. After a while they somehow conned me into going to school there and so I ended up staying for two years. However the place wasn't a home. First and foremost it was an institution; it was run like a hospital. I'd lived a normal life up till then and suddenly I was flung into a ward environment with lots of other girls ranging in age from four to about my age. I had no privacy. I didn't have much to do. And I got depressed. And their solution was to give me antidepressants. I still think that's amazing. I was depressed for a reason, but instead of fixing

317

the circumstances and addressing what was happening in my life, they just gave me pills. After some time they decided I could come off the pills, but when I got a bit down again (I think it was probably just before my period) they just put me straight back on them.

Probably not till ten or fifteen years later did I really do something about the depression. In my outer life I was carrying on okay and I am sure people probably thought I was a confident and happy person, but in my inner self, there was a whole lot more going on. I knew there were reasons for how I felt. I started going to counsellors and psychologists (I was still on antidepressants off and on) and I'd be alright for a while, I'd buck up again, but on a deeper level nothing really changed. The core of me was still frightened and insecure. And then I got to a point when I realised that what I was doing was just surface stuff.

So that's when I decided to undertake psychoanalysis – the 'talking cure'. I spent six years doing that and for the middle four years I went there every weekday. Five days a week. I thought I would never get to the end. The depths are so deep and you really need balls and persistence to continue year after year. I thought I would never be able to live without that psychiatrist. The whole thing about falling in love with your psychiatrist is true . . . but it's just because I transferred everything onto her. But I got through it and if there's anything I'm proud of in my life, I'm proud of that. I might still get frightened, I might still get worried . . . but now I'm no longer frightened in my core.

What was it about psychoanalysis that had such an impact?

I was listening to myself. Day after day, year after year I was listening to my words and I realised I was parroting the world's attitudes and hearing them come out of my own mouth. After a while it started to make me feel sick. I realised it was just crap: 'This is all rubbish, Glenda! This is fantasy land!' I started to see through myself. I was tripping myself up. I could intellectualise everything, but my core didn't believe it. You have to go through tremendous pain to make changes at a core or deeper level rather than just at an intellectual level. People try to avoid that pain.

What do you mean by 'core'?

My core was once like an air pocket into which I'd let other people put their stuff; I'd let other people build my core. But after psychoanalysis I began to see it as something strong like a metal . . . not a hard rigid metal, but a *fluid* metal like mercury. Its fluidity is important, because I don't want to be rigid. The core may also move if I get shoved around a bit, it may get dented, but it no longer breaks. Other people can't put anything into it any more. The core is something I can now depend on. I guess it's about belief in myself. It's about my basic self-esteem. And self-worth. Society has certain attitudes towards people with disabilities and I had soaked up those attitudes just as much as anyone else.

Could you tell me more about those attitudes?

Self-loathing is what it really comes down. It's what I call The Cycle of Negativity . . . if you're born with a disability and if that disability is obvious when you pop out of your mother's womb, the instant reaction to you by everyone around, is one of dismay and sadness. They use words like 'wrong', 'imperfect', 'we'll fix this'. It's negative, negative, negative . . . from the split second you hit that bed . . . and it continues your whole life. It seeps through your psyche and soul and you believe it because that's all you get. And along with that come people's low expectations of you. You're not expected to do your schoolwork. You're not expected to get a job. You're not expected to play sport. You're not even expected to finish your whole drawing in an art lesson . . . and on top of that you're paraded in front of physios and they talk about what's wrong with you and how they're going to fix you. You're put through pain. You're put in callipers. And then on top of your crooked legs and your extraordinarily skinny arms, you feel even uglier than you already are.

Did you feel that the treatment you received was objectifying you in some way?

I don't think it was that bad. Recently I was explaining The Cycle of Negativity to a head of nursing. As I was talking and I watched her face gradually change as she understood its effect on people with disabilities, I suddenly got an insight that was tremendously comforting for me: while all these physios, doctors, parents and whoever else was doing all this negative stuff, it was actually done with the *best* of intentions. They cared and they were trying to help. That helped me to forgive. And yet *how* they did it was still destroying me.

They were doing it in their 'normal' way. They were trying to make me into *them*, because that's all they knew. They believed that their form of normality sort of 'works' in the world. But I'm not them and I never can be them. People with disabilities aren't considered whole. Because of my physical lack, people believe that other parts of my life must be lacking as well.

What does it mean to be treated as a whole person?

It means not ignoring or highlighting any one single aspect.

What does it mean for you personally?

Well that's a hard question for me to answer, because I don't know. In my dreams I sometimes run, but I am running carefully and slowly. I don't know what it's like to really run. I don't know what it's like to be treated as a whole person.

If they could have done something differently at that time, what would it be?

Ask *us* what we thought . . . and accept everybody for who they are . . . accept that they have a whole human being in front of them, whether black, white, able-bodied, crippled, male, female, child, adult, demented . . . there is a reason for every person. If 'Mary' is in a persistent vegetative state, people might think she is entirely useless, but what she provides is the opportunity for someone whose calling it is, to look after her . . . change her urine bag, clean up her shit . . .

Does The Cycle of Negativity also apply to people who have *acquired* a disability?

It applies to people who acquire disabilities later on in life but they already have a basis of self-worth, a basis of expectation of achievement . . . and that will be big or small depending on what point in their lives they acquired their disability. With me, it comes as part of the package. I ingested it my entire life. I will always have to fight it.

In what way does it continue to play a part in your life?

Every day people in society shun me. They are frightened and embarrassed by people with disabilities. For example, if I'm going down the road in my wheelchair, people will cross the road so they don't have to look at me or say hello. Other times they will smile at me with a patronising smile or talk to me like I have an intellectual disability. It is sometimes very hard and even shocking to come to terms with people's prejudices. They have very strange ideas about me. The general population thinks we're trouble. They think we're going to hassle them. They think we're going to cling on to them and hang around. People with disabilities are just like everyone else: they are fabulous, they are no-hopers, they are arse-holes, they are clever ... there's all of us there. If people are with me for a while they will realise that I am just a normal person but with weak muscles. That's all! I have always felt in my soul that I am just as good as anybody else, but the day-to-day stuff always puts me in an inferior position.

You sound as if you've been enormously angry.

Before I started psychoanalysis I had assumed that able-bodied people knew everything, could do everything and that they didn't help me because they didn't care. After psychoanalysis I realised that *no way* did they know everything, *no way* could they do everything and the reason they didn't help me was because they didn't understand me and were ignorant of me. And that was a hugely forgiving point for me to get to. But I've had huge amounts of anger at able-bodied people − ABs, Abes or uprights − because although I was being nice to them, I actually hated them.

Why did you hate them?

Because they had power and control over me ... and that's where the depression comes in. Depression to me is a sense of no control and a lack of some sort of power compared to most people without disabilities. But I also feel I don't have any control over my destiny. When you've got a physical disability, particularly a progressive one, you're at the mercy of your disability. There's a lack of stability and certainty there.

I had a sister who also had spinal muscular atrophy

but she had a more severe form than I do. She was six years older than me and died when she was ten. I was brought up Catholic, and in the last photos I have of my sister she was wearing her First Holy Communion dress. As I reached the age of *my* First Holy Communion I lay in bed at night terrified and I didn't know why. I couldn't have articulated it at the time. Only later did I realise that I had assumed I would *also* die after my First Holy Communion. I had lumped the two together.

You felt you were living under a death threat?

Yes. And I lived under that death threat until I was in my early 40s. Because she died so young and so many of my peers, particularly boys with Duchenne muscular dystrophy, died so young, it was like I also had a hatchet hanging over my head. I was waiting for the thread on which it was hanging to break.

What happened in your early 40s to change that?

I found out that there are three types of spinal muscular atrophy. Type I usually die in infancy, type II live to teens or early adulthood and type III have normal life expectancy. I decided that I must be type III because I wasn't dead yet!

Also, when I was in psychoanalysis I was beginning to understand myself more and come out of the self-loathing. I was also working in disability advocacy at the time and that made me even more knowledgeable about society's attitudes and my own attitudes to myself. I was beginning to throw off these attitudes all over the place. And then I began to talk about having a baby . . .

When I was young they didn't really know anything about these muscle diseases. They didn't know how they were inherited. There is a type of duchenne muscular dystrophy that is definitely carried from mother to son.

I'd met my husband-to-be in my teens, and because of society's attitudes to people like me, I decided at the very young age of seventeen that I should have my tubes tied. I didn't want to 'breed any more of me'. The only 'counselling' I got before making that decision was from a doctor at the hospital, who asked, 'Are you sure?' They had no qualms about sterilising a seventeen-year-old, because I had a disability. They didn't want me breeding any more of me either.

But the thought of having a child came up?

Yes. My husband and I made an appointment to see a geneticist to see if I was a carrier. While I was waiting the six weeks for the results I decided that it would be fine if I *did* have a child with spinal muscular atrophy, because that child would be just like me. I thought, 'Doesn't everybody want a little girl or a little boy just like me!' And that was just such a turning point, because that was accepting *me* and the child I had been. That was the biggest acceptance in my whole life.

With that acceptance of my inner child and therefore myself, I began to accept the fact I'd internalised other people's beliefs about my early demise. I realised that deep inside I had never truly believed that I would die young. But the drawback of realising this, was that rather than a death sentence, I now had a *life* sentence. I felt robbed of a certain self-righteous sookiness; 'Oh shit, now the joke's on me!'

What were the results of the genetic testing?

The geneticist said that my husband and I had no more chance of having a child with spinal muscular atrophy than anybody else. He said that it needed two carriers to come together. He offered to see if I could get the tubal ligation reversed. He rang me a week later to tell me that as a teenager they hadn't just done a tubal ligation . . .

without my consent they had done an irreversible sterili-sation. That was one of the blackest days of my life. I was *supremely* angry and *supremely* sad.

We looked at IVF but in the end we decided not to pursue it. The whole process would have been an onerous one and we also had to consider the impact pregnancy might have on me physically. Also, my husband had been one of ten kids and he wasn't exactly rushing to have children. The important thing was that I got to the point of deciding that I *could* have kids. Whether I had them or not was beside the point.

You mentioned earlier that working in disability advocacy also gave you an understanding of society's attitudes to disability.

When I first started working in advocacy it was as though it was heaven-sent. Someone was actually paying me to help other people complain about disability dis-crimination! For a while I thought I was going to change the world. But however patient I was and however much I tried to change attitudes, I began to understand just how concrete and insidious they were in society.

For example, I had to battle for over two years just to get a waste paper bin removed out of an accessible toilet in a hotel . . . I remember trying to tell the manager of the hotel that the waste paper bin restricted wheel-chair access, but he wouldn't even talk with me. I went to my boss and said, 'I just want to shoot this guy down with a machine gun'. . . . a metaphorical one of course! My boss said, 'Well you've got a better tool than a machine gun, you've got the DDA.'[21] I realised that I didn't just have to battle on my own any more.

. . . but then eventually I got to the point of thinking

---

21 Disability Discrimination Act

that I may as well just get up each morning, stand next to a wall and bang my head against it . . .

In September 1999 I got burnt out. I went into work and just sat at my desk, completely overwhelmed. I wasn't functioning any more. I'd been there for six years and I didn't have anything left in me. I was hiding a lot in marijuana. I got stoned so I didn't have to deal with any of it. And eventually I *had* to break down. I *had* to be suicidal. I *had* to fall in a snivelling heap. I couldn't go on any more. I drove 100 kph down the main road thinking, 'You fuckers! I'll just run the lot of you over.' I was ready to kill anyone who got in my way. I realised that I could not live disability discrimination 24 hours a day in my own life *and* also fight for other people. I knew I needed help.

Did you get that help?

My husband and I went to the hospital so I could be admitted. My psychiatrist/psychoanalyst was able to get me into a brand new psychiatric ward that should have been accessible.

We sat down and we told them why we were there. I told them that I was supremely angry about discrimination and I told them what my needs were in relationship to my disability. An hour and a half later they told me that the accessible room had already been taken. We were shown down a long corridor to another room. Along the way they pointed out a window where I could get my medication. It was far above my head. I was already supremely angry and I could see they had ignored a lot of access issues. I started to get even angrier.

They showed me to my room and they opened the door and the bed stuck out so far that I could not have accessed the bathroom. I got even angrier, so they turned the bed around. There were no rails . . . there was nothing in the bathroom. I started ramming their brand new paintwork with my wheelchair. This went on for a while. My husband was getting stressed too. He had just about had it with me and everything else that was going on. We were arguing with the staff about the access issues and they were being quite cocky. That only enraged me further.

People started gathering in the hallway to watch as though we were some sort of sideshow. My husband said, 'Get all these people away!' He went up to some double doors to shut them against the throng of people, but because they were fire doors they slammed shut loudly. I could see that the staff thought he was getting violent. At some stage my husband came back in the room and said, 'I think we'd better go, they're threatening to detain both of us.' Rather than see our anger as justified, they only saw it as a reason to commit us both. We went out in the hallway and we saw two security guards with rubber gloves coming towards us . . . we literally fled the hospital . . . at nine o'clock on a cold rainy night . . . Later I was admitted to the veterans' hospital.

Was that an improvement?

My psychiatrist happened to work at the veteran's hospital and she said she could get me in at the old soldiers' hospital. I said, 'Well I'm an old soldier aren't I!' and she said, 'Yes you are.' And that was like manna from heaven. It was the only time in the whole of psychoanalysis that she said something *real* to me. It was recognition and acknowledgment. I stayed there for a month.

While I was there I remember thinking, 'Who would understand what it's like to have what I have . . . depression, my worries, my life? The Vietnam veterans!' It's obviously not the same . . . but they went away to war.

They went through horrors that we cannot imagine. They came back from that and they were shunned, spat at and vilified. And now they're mentally ill because of it. They can't get rid of the pictures in their heads, they can't get rid of their experiences . . . it continues every day. But that was a really fabulous time. I shared a lot with the vets. We'd talk about, 'Who's really mad? We may be in here, but look at all them out there!'

It sounds as though the camaraderie was important.

Yes. 'Them out there' were the *really* crazy ones. There is an arrogance about *them*. They believe that they are the 'right' human beings as opposed to the hobos and the cripples and the mentally ill. They feel that they are the genuine article and yet they don't know how much they are actually crippled by that belief. It gets in their way because they never search beyond that . . .

Was the vets' hospital accessible?

Because I was angry and I was an advocate for people with disabilities and because I knew that things were supposed to be accessible for *all* people, I stuck stickers on things that said *Inaccessible/Unacceptable*. I stuck them on the phone, the café bar, next to the light switches, on the toilet, on the front and back doors. I let them know in no uncertain terms. A couple of the vets plaited some ropes and attached them to the door handles so that I could open them more easily, but the staff took them off. They were planning a ward refurbishment and they had plans up on the wall for people to comment on so I made some suggestions.

Did they follow them up?

Four years later I once again dropped my bundle and I went back there . . . I needed a little rest again. They had refurbished the place but hadn't made it any more accessible for a person in a wheelchair. Apparently you can't have two disabilities. If you've got depression you can't have a physical disability. None of the advice I had given them on my previous visit had been put into practice.

On my second night there, my bed malfunctioned and I had to sleep on a steep slope all night. I woke up exhausted and in such pain. At breakfast time they put my tray the wrong way around and I asked them to turn it around and the nurse said, 'You wouldn't want us to be doing things for you that you could do yourself, would you?' I wasn't in there for physical rehabilitation! It was double discrimination. They knew on the ward that I was very independent and wouldn't have asked for help unless I needed it. I had needed mental and physical rest, but being on the ward that second time only exacerbated things both mentally and physically. I discharged myself a few days later and put in a complaint under the DDA.

So you never really got the care and the rest you needed in any of the facilities?

In the end . . . not even in the vets' hospital. The very first time was okay because I was more physically able . . .

What about general psychiatric care?

Not a hell of a lot. What I got out of being in hospital was what I shared with the vets and what they shared with me . . . and some physical rest. Some anger management stuff was good and I had some time to think.

Were you put on medication?

They put me on medication when I was in there four years previously. An antidepressant. They put me on a high dose. About a year later I was still on it and I started getting terrible neck cramps that forced my chin down onto my chest. Unless I held my head completely upright it would snap down. Over a period of several months these cramps greatly reduced my already limited walking ability. I went to the doctor and she suggested that I go to a physio. Then I got urgency incontinence and so I got some pills for that. Anyway, after a while I wondered whether the antidepressant could be causing my problems, so I got on the Internet and looked up its side effects. Sure enough . . . muscle weakness, neck cramps and urgency incontinence! They shouldn't have given that drug to someone who has only ten per cent of average muscle strength! . . . and urgency incontinence! I'm in a wheelchair and of course I was wetting myself! I went to my doctor and she said, 'Oh you shouldn't have been on such a high dose for so long.' My doctor and my psychiatrist had both seriously fucked up. I lost an enormous amount of muscle strength during that time and I probably won't get it back. If I didn't need my doctor and psychiatrist I would probably sue them.

What is your overall opinion on the use of medication for depression?

Pills certainly help, but on the whole it is just a medical quick fix. It does nothing to fix the core or the cause of the problem. People are hassled and sad, lonely and struggling. There are so many reasons to be depressed. I don't believe that I'm actually a depressed person. I believe that I'm happy and strong but I'm not fucking superwoman! If you look at that scale of trauma in just the last four-year period . . . divorce, job loss, death of my parents and coping with a disability . . . so to say I just need pills is so demeaning of my coping capabilities, which are huge! But I think part of the problem is also that we live in this false world in which people try to present as beautiful and wonderful and having sex three times a week. Nobody's doing that and yet part of us believes we have to match up to that picture. The way I look at antidepressants is that they lighten the load for a little while. That's all. I would prefer not to depend on drugs.

Are you taking medication now?

I came off that antidepressant and I was okay for a few months, but then I got depressed again. I went to my psychiatrist for another sort of antidepressant but the urinary incontinence started again. I can't move fast and so I'd either wet myself or I'd have to use pads. I'm living in poverty as it is and I can't afford the extra expense of pads. Then I went to my doctor and she said these pills were of the same class as the original ones. I wondered why my psychiatrist had given them to me! My doctor gave me something else and then in three or four days I was vomiting and had diarrhoea. The doctor said it was probably just a gastro bug . . . I stopped taking them.

Do you still get support from your psychiatrist?

I'm not getting a lot from my psychiatrist any more. I can tell her things I can't tell anyone else. She listens to me. I get sympathy and understanding from her. Sometimes she just gives me little strategies to deal with life, but right now I have no *refuge*. I can't go to hospital because it's inaccessible. Friends' houses are inaccessible. On top of that there's no money for more support hours at the moment. My wheelchair cushion has exacerbated the curve on my spine and I've been waiting eighteen months for a new cushion. I got a letter the other day, telling me that there was no more money for support hours and they gave me two alternatives: to go into a group or cluster home, for which there is a long waiting list, or to go into a nursing home. I'm 48 and I'm *not* going to live in a nursing home. So that's where I am. Depressed.

Over time has the way you experience that depression changed?

My depression before psychoanalysis was frightened. I'm not frightened through to my core any more. I certainly get frightened in my mind or outer shell, but I stay solid in my core. And I feel I can *do* something about my depression now. I am not as much at its mercy. The things I can't do anything about, the things I can't change, like my disability, don't sadden or depress me any more.

In a way I see depression as accumulative. If you have to keep walking forever, your legs will start to ache. Eventually though, you'll get really tired and fall down. You fall down and you'll have a rest because you simply can't get up. It's like that with the mental stuff as well. Depression is the falling down. The exhaustion. That's where I am at the moment.

Do you feel that in essence the depression is *making* you rest?

Certainly not in the past, but right now it is. I think that whatever it is that I'm supposed to be doing can just get stuffed. I'm not *able* to do it. I've got this voluntary work to do but I just want to sit and watch Oprah on telly. And this time I'm saying to myself, 'It's okay Glenda. You're *allowed* to. Look at all you have to cope with . . . deaths, divorce, disability. Look at all you have to do in just one day. Give it a rest!' I don't *want* to sit and watch Oprah all day, but if that's where I'm at, then I'll give myself permission to do that.

And how does it feel to give yourself that permission?

Quite powerful. I can get quite anxious about it, because I am a doer and a worker . . . but now that I'm allowing myself to be depressed, I'm recognising how hard I do work and am no longer pushing myself to be 'normal'. I'm recognising that I am only 'Miss Ten Percent' in the physical world and that's okay.

You see yourself as 'Miss Ten Percent' in terms of physical strength. How do see yourself in mental, emotional, spiritual or intellectual terms?

Having overcome tremendous mental and emotional struggle, and this sounds a bit immodest, I actually think I'm *better* than the average bear! If an able-bodied person does weight lifting, he or she will probably be 110 per cent compared to the average person. All my life I've had to undergo emotional weight training. I've had to push against some enormous emotional negatives, even maintaining the sheer conviction that I am 100 per cent of a person in the face of the world telling me that I'm not. I know I'm strong. I've always been quick-thinking and intelligent, but because I owned the 'second-class citizen' thing for such a long time I just didn't allow myself to truly embody those qualities.

Sir Edmund Hilary climbed Mt Everest and got medals and fame and fortune. By midday Joe Blow with quadriplegia has probably got out of bed and had a shower, and yet that's *his* Mt Everest. But nobody's ever going to say to him, 'Well done, Joe!' . . . nobody's ever going to give him a medal! . . . In fact they're more likely to criticise him. The emotional strength I require to simply get my jumper on . . . I could get enraged by the effort that's required . . . but I can't do that, because I'd be enraged the entire time. But that emotional control and patience and perseverance is just *huge*! And the fears I've had to overcome . . . of falling over with every step. When people don't have anything to overcome in their lives they just become wimps!

So the struggle has brought enormous strength . . .

. . . and understanding. Through all my experiences I've come to understand that nobody is different to anybody else. Through the struggle with myself and against my hate of able-bodied people, I've realised that everybody struggles. Some people who appear to have everything struggle even more than I do. I realise I am not special. It's been humbling in a way. When I get depressed or I think people aren't helping me, I think, 'Well *they're* actually struggling too.' I'm not worse off than anybody else. I never thought I'd be able to say that. I'm a lot kinder on myself. I don't have to be super woman or super crip any more!

Appendix A

Further notes on language and technical details

- It is important to make the distinction between psychiatrists who focus primarily on diagnosis and medication and those who have obtained further specialist training in psychotherapy or psychoanalysis. The latter have competency in the former but the former does not necessarily imply competency in the latter. The terms 'prescribing psychiatrists', 'psychiatrists in the system', 'consultant psychiatrists' or 'public psychiatrists' are used to indicate the former. In the case of the latter, the distinction is clearly made in the course of the interview. Glenda mentions that her psychiatrist also practises psychoanalysis. Joan states that her psychiatrist is also a psychotherapist.
- I asked each interviewee to provide some material for the beginning of the interview: a photo, something about why the photo was important and then a short introduction that at the very least included the interviewee's name and age. I suggested that this material might draw the reader into the body of the

interview. Most interviewees gave a great deal of thought to their photos, whether of themselves or something that 'spoke' of who they are as people. Some interviewees wished their diagnosis/diagnoses included, others felt that this was not important for an understanding of who they are. Wayne makes this particularly clear in his opening description.

- Many interviewees had an opinion about the use of the words 'mental illness'. Many felt they were inadequate or inappropriate in any discussion of their felt suffering or lives. Many make this quite clear in the course of their interview (see Appendix B). Any use of these words (or for that matter *any* words) in quotation marks is at the request of the interviewee themselves. Because of their questionable nature for many of interviewees, I have also decided to put the words 'mental illness' in quotation marks in the subtitle of the book, the introduction and the appendices. I hope that in doing so it will not only give acknowledgment to the interviewees but also give readers some pause before accepting wholesale their general meanings and the accompanying assumptions.

- My intention in using the interview format was that a dialogue would have a freshness and spontaneity that would be real and personal. I hoped that this would bring out the humanity, but also the unique character and personality of the interviewees. However, the drawback to this was that spoken English does not always read easily on the page. I often had to walk a fine line in my editing processes: I had to make the interviews readable while not destroying their essential character and personal appeal.

- Some interviewees spoke in the second person
  singular for quite large sections – 'you' instead of 'I'.
  Although quite common in spoken English, this can
  become rather unwieldy in written English. In my
  process of editing the interviews, I had to be aware of
  readability while not losing sight of the fact that
  speaking in the second person singular may indicate a
  certain detachment. Generally I made a decision to
  leave *some* second person singular in the interview
  when it did not impact on overall readability. Those
  interviews in which there is no second person
  singular present are accurate in their representation.
- A couple of interviewees presented me with large
  tracts of written material after the first interview.
  I opted at no stage to use any of this material, citing
  my desire for spontaneity and immediacy.
- If a very strong mood or feeling was present in the
  spoken English but was not necessarily evident on
  reading, I generally chose to reflect this mood.
  For instance when Patrick speaks of the people he
  met while homeless, I reflect, '. . . you speak of those
  people with great fondness.'
- I have added ellipsis points (. . .) to indicate a
  natural hiatus in the flow of speech of the
  interviewee. This can imply a period of concentrated
  thought, a tangible reliving of an incident, or an
  attempt to find the right words. In my questions
  ellipsis points indicate that I was interrupted.
- As mentioned in the introduction, I felt that
  my questions should not be interrogative or
  confrontational in any way. I felt that my questions
  should be simple and merely promote the natural
  flow of the interviewees' rhythm and story. I *very*
  much tailored my questions to suit each individual

interviewee. Questions I may have asked of one interviewee didn't necessarily imply that I might ask a similar question of another. At times I was silent and felt no need to interrupt. At other times interviewees, such as Leah, responded well to more intense questioning.

- Only four interviewees, David, Dimitri, Eva and Meg chose not to use their real names. Some names within the interviews may be pseudonyms. All pseudonyms are used at the request of the interviewee.
- All quotations are used at the request of the interviewee.

Appendix B

Some general points of agreement between
interviews

- The vast majority of those interviewed had sought
  help from the **public mental health system** at some
  time. Although the services it had provided had kept
  people alive in difficult circumstances, it was
  generally not the mental health system and its use of
  the medical model, that had brought about healing or
  understanding.
- In writing of **psychiatrists** it is important to make the
  distinction between psychiatrists who have had
  further training in psychotherapy or psychoanalysis
  and those who have not (*see* Appendix A). In
  describing the latter the general summation was,
  'They just prescribed medication' (Leah). With
  regard to the former, an overwhelming majority of
  interviewees spoke of the value of 'talking therapies'
  and the importance of a **long-term relationship
  with a therapist**. This therapist could be a
  counsellor, psychotherapist, psychiatrist or
  psychologist by profession. The general consensus was

that it was necessary to go outside the system to obtain this sort of help.

- **Key workers** within the system were seen by a number of interviewees as important and helpful, primarily because a longer term and more intimate relationship was possible.
- A number of interviewees spoke of being subject to difficult or catch-22 situations in their treatment by the mental health system. As Cheryl sums up:

> I knew I had to play the game to get what I needed.

- Most people interviewed had experienced some sort of **trauma** in their lives and saw this as giving rise to the suffering that was subsequently termed 'mental illness'. This trauma was mostly in the form of child abuse or childhood difficulty but also included the death of children (David and Coralie), the death of a spouse (Coralie), divorce/disability/death (Glenda) and the break up of relationships. Some felt that in the light of this trauma, the words 'mental illness' were inadequate or even wrong. Patrick states:

> I just want to say at this point that I don't believe there is such a thing as 'mental illness'. I prefer to call it mental trauma. I think the stigma attached to the words 'mental illness' is too difficult to remove. It becomes embedded in you like a virus and you can't get rid of it.

and also Eva:

> I think you *need* to ask what 'mental illness' actually is ... I think most 'mental illness' is what happens to a human being who has been traumatised and has not

had the resources either inside or outside to understand what has happened ... People aren't 'mentally ill' ... they're traumatised!

- Many felt that there was no acknowledgment by the mental health system of the **devastating impact of childhood trauma and abuse**. Joan spoke of this:

> During my years in the mental health service I picked up very clearly that there is a *big* taboo in declaring that your parents played a large part in the creation of your so-called 'mental illness'.

- For many it was significant that being diagnosed and labelled with a 'mental illness' carried with it an associated **stigma**. Cheryl comments:

> At the clinic I hear people talking about integrating people with 'mental illness' into society, but by definition of what they have done, they have made that impossible. They label you as 'mentally ill', and then push you back into a society that thinks, 'Oh my god, "*mental illness*"!'

- In the light of dehumanising treatment many interviews contain an implicit plea to be treated as a **human being**. Many define what it is to be a human being.
- A few interviewees questioned the use of the word '**depression**'. They believed that 'breakdown' or even 'breakthrough' was a more accurate terminology. Glenda and Dimitri both saw depression as a process which they felt it necessary to follow. In respect to this, Dimitri speaks of articles he had read which he subsequently applied in his own life:

The basic approach of the articles was that depression was something that was actually beneficial if you could accept it and go through it, even if wasn't necessarily comfortable; that depression was a deepening process during which a lot of the questions and notions you had about yourself and about life needed to be taken in deeply and felt, rather than just thought about and questioned.

- Many spoke highly of the importance of **friendship** and the honesty, compassion, support, perseverance, love, communication, understanding, acceptance and connection it brought. A number spoke of the importance of camaraderie during hospitalisations. This is summed up by Cheryl:

   > Rather than the psychiatrists or the medications it was my interactions with other patients that informed my behaviour and helped me.

   and also Linda:

   > It was all of us, the so-called 'mentally ill', who were the therapy. We did our own therapy by talking with one another.

   Overall, it was **relationship** and connection, whether with professionals or with friends and family, that were seen as paramount. John says:
   > ... I recognised from this episode, that if you go to a psychiatrist, it's the *need to relate* that's most important ... that's what matters.

- The importance of **listening** was highlighted in the introduction. Further to those comments, people were in agreement that in order to be 'listened' to and to get the treatment that was needed within the system it was sometimes necessary to 'act out'. Eva, Coralie and Trevor mention this.

- Although **medication** was seen by many as necessary, the negative consequences and repercussions outweighed the good. Glenda sums up:

> Pills certainly help, but on the whole it is just a medical quick fix. It does nothing to fix the core or the cause of the problem.

Almost all interviewees suffered **side effects** from medication, some of which were quite devastating. Some people had sustained irreversible side effects. These included muscle wastage (Glenda) and a rotting liver (Coralie). The many shorter-term side effects had also affected people's lives considerably. There was also a general consensus that psychiatrists minimised, invalidated, denied or ascribed the impact of side effects to different causes.

- Most interviewees spoke of their **lack of identity or sense of self** as being the major causative factor to their suffering. This was seen by most as resulting from a childhood of abuse or difficulty. This lack of a sense of self was described in many different ways: of having no 'I' or 'me', not being at home, not having a voice, having no self-esteem, being a 'nothing', emptiness, having no core solidity, 'poor little bugger inside', etc. Often the treatment by the mental health system only exacerbated the sense that people felt they were 'nothing'. Several experienced the treatment they had received, both in and out of hospital, as re-traumatising and similar to that which they had experienced in their childhoods. Although all agreed that there were good people within the system there were many stories of disdainful and unenlightened treatment.

- Many interviewees highlighted the importance of a **spiritual context** when coming to a sense of lasting peace, contentment or healing within their lives. This context was given many different names including that of Christianity, God, spirit and/or soul. Wayne speaks of reclaiming his Aboriginal heritage and as such also his spiritual connection to the land and to the natural world around him.

- A number of interviewees spoke of their suffering in terms of **deeper philosophical and life questions** for which they wanted answers. As Christie says:

> I had always had all these searching questions about the meaning of life but I'd just never asked them or when I did ask them, people would say, 'You think too much, that's your problem.' They were questions like: What's really important? What happens after we die? How can all these bad things be happening in the world?

- Several interviewees felt that their suffering was highly **meaningful**. Cheryl says:

> I felt it was *all* meaningful. I felt that there was a reason for it *all*. Something was driving me. I had an overwhelming sense of being driven by 'something'. But I didn't know yet what that meaning or reason was.

Several felt that their violence, 'acting out' and self-harm were also meaningful but not generally seen as such. Coralie says:

> People are trying to manage the experience of trauma when they're acting out, they're trying to communicate and once you break through that they'll stop acting out.

- A number of interviewees spoke of their **suffering in positive terms**. Meg says:

> Suffering is a horrible thing at the time but I think the pay-off for that is that you live a much fuller life. And a deeper life. And you can connect with other people better. There are many positive things that come out of suffering.

and John:

> My discovery that many of the great spiritual writers – including Mother Teresa of Calcutta – say that suffering is a gift was a great joy to me . . . it hit me between the eyes! It makes it so much easier to accept the road that I've travelled down. Suffering can seem to be so negative yet it can, if we allow it, produce in our Being the positive gift of compassion. Compassion doesn't come out of thin air.

- Many spoke of understanding their lives and suffering in terms of a '**journey**' or an adventure. When asked what the metaphor of a journey had brought to her life, Sarah replied:

It's about coming to a sense of peace, of understanding and of accepting my life wherever I'm at and wherever it takes me. If I deal with what I have at that time in the best way I possibly can, with the resources that are around me or with the resources that I have within, then I'll continue on the journey.

- **Creativity** was an important aspect of the lives of a number of interviewees. This could be painting (Joan), music (Meg and David), writing (Meg and Trevor), film (Dimitri) or craft work (Linda and Joan). Patrick and Christie spoke of life itself as being a creative process.
- Three interviewees (George, Linda and Eva) mentioned the **Second World War** and the impact it had had on their parents' lives and as such also on them as children. George had also lived through the war as a small child.
- The **media** and the 'perfect' world it portrayed was seen by many as having a negative impact. When asked what he put the high incidence of depression down to, George answered:

> The media. The continual watching of violence on the TV. The anxiety of 'you've got to have this, you've got to have that, you've got to be good looking, you can't be fat'. People tend to overlook the good things about themselves.

Some people also commented that they felt the portrayal of the 'mentally ill' in the media was inaccurate. Linda says:

The media portray the 'mentally ill' as violent. But the truth is that we'd much rather kill *ourselves* than anybody else. I apologise to an ant or a spider if I kill it. I don't want to hurt anybody or anything.

- A number of interviewees spoke of the importance and need for a place of **sanctuary or refuge** that was apart from hospitalisation and assessment and apart from the difficulties of everyday life. This could be a 'safe space', silence, home or an actual place of refuge.
- Several interviewees spoke of the value of **animals** in their lives.

Wakefield Press is an independent publishing and
distribution company based in Adelaide, South Australia.
We love good stories and publish beautiful books.
To see our full range of titles, please visit our website at
www.wakefieldpress.com.au.